MY IBD JOURNAL

The information in this work is provided for educational purposes only. It is not a substitute for consultation with a trained medical practitioner. Please consult your physician before beginning, changing, or discontinuing any healthcare regimen.

This journal is dedicated to my mother and father Connie and Andy, my siblings Ashlyn and Matt, my cousin and best friend Justin and my closest friends the Luths. You have all helped me to be who I am today.

CONTENTS

PREFACE A PERSONAL STORY

I don't think I need to be philosophical here to tell my story, or for you to realize the impact that IBD has on your life. Most likely, you've chosen to purchase this journal because you yourself suffer from some form of IBD. Personally, I suffer from Crohn's and have for the past six years.

Most recently, I chose to create this journal due to some unfortunate events in my life which included a small bowel resection that led to six weeks of bed rest, and for awhile, an unknown future. Put simply, I ignored the signs, mismanaged my disease, and did not follow doctor's orders, which led to appetite loss, weight loss, swollen joints, fatigue, mental strain, and finally intestinal blockage, which resulted in surgery.

With my recent surgery, I cannot say that this year has not been a challenge for me. However, this challenge forced me to face many personal obstacles that I feel were holding me back from achieving my full potential, both personally and professionally. Since my surgery, I have pro-actively pursued a healthy lifestyle, professional development, and a deeper relationship with God. I have chosen to rise above IBD by acknowledging that it exists and facing it head on rather than ignoring it. Doing so has proven rewarding.

My hopes are that you will use this journal to do the same in your life and subsequently reap the rewards of your effort. Take the time necessary to truly manage your disease and track your health, then take this journal with you to each doctor visit and use it to recall and share anything you may want to talk about with your doctor. Prevention is on the other side of life's door; you are the key.

Be Blessed,
Ryan Kral

Note: In the back of this journal you will find helpful tools to track foods, medicines, and your family tree.

Did you know?: Creating a detailed history of family members who have had any medical conditions can help your doctor to correctly asses medications that should be prescribed. Use the Family Tree example diagram in the back of this journal to map out any family members with any known medical conditions.

DAY 001

📅 **Date** _____

🌡️ **Temperature** _____   ⚖️ **Weight** _____

💊 **Medications Taken Today**

1 _____   2 _____   3 _____

🩹 **Pain** (Circle most painful moment)

0 — 1 — 2 — 3 — 4 — 5 — 6 — 7 — 8 — 9 — **10**

GOOD   BAD

Types of Pain (circle all that apply)

| DULL | THROBBING | SHARP | CRAMPING |

How long did the pain last? (circle the longest time)

0 1 2 3 4 5 6 7 8 9 10 11 12 13 14 15 16 17 18 19 20 [More +]

Minutes

How many times have you experienced pain today? _____

⚡ **Sickness Symptoms** (cough, sweats, feel cold, loss of appetite)

_____

🚽 **Bowel Movements** (bowel movement scale: 1 = Loose // 6 = Hard)

BM #1 ① ② 3 4 5 6   BM #3 ① ② 3 4 5 6

BM #2 ① ② 3 4 5 6   BM #4 ① ② 3 4 5 6

BM Notes _____

🩺 **Do you need to call your doctor?**   [YES]   [NO]

1

Ⓒ **Breakfast** _____

_____

Ⓢ **Snack** _____

_____

▢ **Lunch** _____

_____

Ⓢ **Snack** _____

_____

🐔 **Dinner** _____

_____

Ⓔ **Exercise** _____ 🕐 **Time Spent Exercising** _____

✅ **What is one good thing that happened today?**

_____

📌 **What can you do to improve tomorrow?**

_____

📋 **Personal Journal / Notes** (write something about your day or personal thoughts)

_____

_____

_____

_____

_____

_____

_____

Tip: If you have a child with IBD, remember that it may be difficult for them to talk about some of their symptoms. Help them to find creative ways to stay on top of their disease by suggesting blogging, journaling, keeping a diary, finding a confidant, or any other means of recording or reporting their condition.

DAY 002

Date _____

Temperature _____   **Weight** _____

Medications Taken Today

1 _____   2 _____   3 _____

Pain (Circle most painful moment)

0　1　2　3　4　5　6　7　8　9　10
GOOD　　　　　　　　　　　　　　　BAD

Types of Pain (circle all that apply)

DULL　　THROBBING　　SHARP　　CRAMPING

How long did the pain last? (circle the longest time)

0　1　2　3　4　5　6　7　8　9　10　11　12　13　14　15　16　17　18　19　20　More +

Minutes

How many times have you experienced pain today? _____

Sickness Symptoms (cough, sweats, feel cold, loss of appetite)

_____

Bowel Movements (bowel movement scale: 1 = Loose // 6 = Hard)

BM #1　1　2　3　4　5　6　　　BM #3　1　2　3　4　5　6

BM #2　1　2　3　4　5　6　　　BM #4　1　2　3　4　5　6

BM Notes _____

Do you need to call your doctor?　YES　　NO

Breakfast ▶_____

_____

Snack ▶_____

_____

Lunch ▶_____

_____

Snack ▶_____

_____

Dinner ▶_____

_____

Exercise ▶_____ 🕐 Time Spent Exercising ▶_____

✔ What is one good thing that happened today?

▶_____

+1 What can you do to improve tomorrow?

▶_____

Personal Journal / Notes (write something about your day or personal thoughts)

▶_____

_____

_____

_____

_____

_____

_____

_____

DAY 003

📅 Date _____

🌡 Temperature _____ 👁 Weight _____

💊 **Medications Taken Today**

1 _____   2 _____   3 _____

✚ **Pain** (Circle most painful moment)

0 — 1 — 2 — 3 — 4 — 5 — 6 — 7 — 8 — 9 — 10

GOOD   BAD

Types of Pain (circle all that apply)

| DULL | THROBBING | SHARP | CRAMPING |

How long did the pain last? (circle the longest time)

0 1 2 3 4 5 6 7 8 9 10 11 12 13 14 15 16 17 18 19 20 [More +]

Minutes

How many times have you experienced pain today? _____

⚡ **Sickness Symptoms** (cough, sweats, feel cold, loss of appetite)

_____

🚽 **Bowel Movements** (bowel movement scale: 1 = Loose // 6 = Hard)

BM #1 ① ② ③ 4 5 6   BM #3 ① ② ③ 4 5 6

BM #2 ① ② ③ 4 5 6   BM #4 ① ② ③ 4 5 6

BM Notes _____

🩺 **Do you need to call your doctor?** | YES | | NO |

5

Breakfast _____
_____

Snack _____
_____

Lunch _____
_____

Snack _____
_____

Dinner _____
_____

Exercise _____   Time Spent Exercising _____

What is one good thing that happened today?
_____

What can you do to improve tomorrow?
_____

Personal Journal / Notes (write something about your day or personal thoughts)
_____
_____
_____
_____
_____
_____
_____

⊕ Tip: Try an avocado—This fruit is full of good fats, B vitamins, vitamin E, and soluble, as well as insoluble fiber.

DAY 004

📅 Date _____

🌡 Temperature _____   ⚖ Weight _____

💊 **Medications Taken Today**

1 _____   2 _____   3 _____

Pain (Circle most painful moment)

⓪ ① ② ③ ④ ⑤ ⑥ ⑦ ⑧ ⑨ ⑩

GOOD   BAD

Types of Pain (circle all that apply)

| DULL | THROBBING | SHARP | CRAMPING |

How long did the pain last? (circle the longest time)

0 1 2 3 4 5 6 7 8 9 10 11 12 13 14 15 16 17 18 19 20 [More +]

Minutes

How many times have you experienced pain today? _____

⚡ **Sickness Symptoms** (cough, sweats, feel cold, loss of appetite)

[   ]

Bowel Movements (bowel movement scale: 1 = Loose // 6 = Hard)

BM #1   ① ② ③ ④ ⑤ ⑥   BM #3   ① ② ③ ④ ⑤ ⑥

BM #2   ① ② ③ ④ ⑤ ⑥   BM #4   ① ② ③ ④ ⑤ ⑥

BM Notes _____

🩺 **Do you need to call your doctor?**   [YES]   [NO]

7

○ **Breakfast** _____

_____

○ **Snack** _____

_____

▢ **Lunch** _____

_____

○ **Snack** _____

_____

○○ **Dinner** _____

_____

○○ **Exercise** _____ ○ **Time Spent Exercising** _____

✓ **What is one good thing that happened today?**

_____

⚑ **What can you do to improve tomorrow?**

_____

▤ **Personal Journal / Notes** (write something about your day or personal thoughts)

_____

_____

_____

_____

_____

_____

_____

⊕ Famous People with IBD: Matt Light, a former American football offensive tackle for the New England Patriots.

📅 **Date** _____

DAY 005

🌡️ **Temperature** _____ 👁️ **Weight** _____

💊 **Medications Taken Today**

1 _____ 2 _____ 3 _____

Pain (Circle most painful moment)

⓪ ① ② ③ ④ ⑤ ⑥ ⑦ ⑧ ⑨ ⑩
GOOD   BAD

Types of Pain (circle all that apply)

| DULL | THROBBING | SHARP | CRAMPING |

How long did the pain last? (circle the longest time)

0 1 2 3 4 5 6 7 8 9 10 11 12 13 14 15 16 17 18 19 20 [More +]
Minutes

How many times have you experienced pain today? _____

⚡ **Sickness Symptoms** (cough, sweats, feel cold, loss of appetite)

_____

Bowel Movements (bowel movement scale: 1 = Loose // 6 = Hard)

BM #1 ① ② ③ 4 5 6   BM #3 ① ② ③ 4 5 6

BM #2 ① ② ③ 4 5 6   BM #4 ① ② ③ 4 5 6

BM Notes _____

🩺 **Do you need to call your doctor?** | YES | | NO |

9

○ **Breakfast** ▶ _____
_____

◎ **Snack** ▶ _____
_____

▢ **Lunch** ▶ _____
_____

◎ **Snack** ▶ _____
_____

Dinner ▶ _____
_____

Exercise ▶ _____ ◷ **Time Spent Exercising** ▶ _____

✔ **What is one good thing that happened today?**

▶ _____

What can you do to improve tomorrow?

▶ _____

▤ **Personal Journal / Notes** (write something about your day or personal thoughts)

▶ _____
_____
_____
_____
_____
_____
_____

⊕ Famous People with IBD: Ben Morrison, famous stand-up comedian and actor.

📅 **Date** _____

DAY 006

🌡️ **Temperature** _____   ⚖️ **Weight** _____

💊 **Medications Taken Today**

1 _____   2 _____   3 _____

Pain (Circle most painful moment)

0 — 1 — 2 — 3 — 4 — 5 — 6 — 7 — 8 — 9 — (10)
GOOD   BAD

Types of Pain (circle all that apply)

DULL | THROBBING | SHARP | CRAMPING

How long did the pain last? (circle the longest time)

0 1 2 3 4 5 6 7 8 9 10 11 12 13 14 15 16 17 18 19 20 More +
Minutes

How many times have you experienced pain today? _____

⚡ **Sickness Symptoms** (cough, sweats, feel cold, loss of appetite)

_____

Bowel Movements (bowel movement scale: 1 = Loose // 6 = Hard)

BM #1 ① ② ③ 4 5 6   BM #3 ① ② ③ 4 5 6

BM #2 ① ② ③ 4 5 6   BM #4 ① ② ③ 4 5 6

BM Notes _____

🩺 **Do you need to call your doctor?**   YES   NO

○○ Breakfast ▶_____

_____

☺ Snack ▶_____

_____

□ Lunch ▶_____

_____

☺ Snack ▶_____

_____

🍗 Dinner ▶_____

_____

○─○ Exercise ▶_____ ⏱ Time Spent Exercising ▶_____

✓ What is one good thing that happened today?

▶_____

➕1 What can you do to improve tomorrow?

▶_____

▤ **Personal Journal / Notes** (write something about your day or personal thoughts)

▶_____

_____

_____

_____

_____

_____

_____

📅 **Date** ▲_____

DAY 007

🌡 **Temperature** ▲_____   👁 **Weight** ▲_____

💊 **Medications Taken Today**

1 ▲_____   2 ▲_____   3 ▲_____

Pain (Circle most painful moment)

0 — 1 — 2 — 3 — 4 — 5 — 6 — 7 — 8 — 9 — 10
GOOD   BAD

Types of Pain (circle all that apply)

| DULL | THROBBING | SHARP | CRAMPING |

How long did the pain last? (circle the longest time)

0 1 2 3 4 5 6 7 8 9 10 11 12 13 14 15 16 17 18 19 20 [More +]
Minutes

How many times have you experienced pain today? ▲_____

⚡ **Sickness Symptoms** (cough, sweats, feel cold, loss of appetite)

_____

Bowel Movements (bowel movement scale: 1 = Loose // 6 = Hard)

BM #1 ① ② ③ 4 5 6   BM #3 ① ② ③ 4 5 6
BM #2 ① ② ③ 4 5 6   BM #4 ① ② ③ 4 5 6

BM Notes ▲_____

🩺 **Do you need to call your doctor?**   YES   NO

13

〇⊃ **Breakfast** ▶—————————————————————————

◔ **Snack** ▶—————————————————————————

⬜ **Lunch** ▶—————————————————————————

◔ **Snack** ▶—————————————————————————

🎧 **Dinner** ▶—————————————————————————

◻–◻ **Exercise** ▶———————— ⏱ **Time Spent Exercising** ▶————————

✔ **What is one good thing that happened today?**

▶—————————————————————————

◀ **What can you do to improve tomorrow?**

▶—————————————————————————

▤ **Personal Journal / Notes** (write something about your day or personal thoughts)

▶—————————————————————————

—————————————————————————

—————————————————————————

—————————————————————————

—————————————————————————

—————————————————————————

⊕ Did you know?: Red bumps, called erythema nodosum, can appear on the shin or ankles and are more common in women than men. For people with IBD, these commonly occur just before or during a flare.

📅 **Date** _____

DAY 008

🌡 **Temperature** _____ ⚖ **Weight** _____

💊 **Medications Taken Today**

1 _____ 2 _____ 3 _____

Pain (Circle most painful moment)

0 — 1 — 2 — 3 — 4 — 5 — 6 — 7 — 8 — 9 — (10)
GOOD   BAD

Types of Pain (circle all that apply)

| DULL | THROBBING | SHARP | CRAMPING |

How long did the pain last? (circle the longest time)

0 1 2 3 4 5 6 7 8 9 10 11 12 13 14 15 16 17 18 19 20 |More +|
Minutes

How many times have you experienced pain today? ▸ _____

⚡ **Sickness Symptoms** (cough, sweats, feel cold, loss of appetite)

_____

🫙 **Bowel Movements** (bowel movement scale: 1 = Loose // 6 = Hard)

BM #1 ① ② ③ 4 5 6   BM #3 ① ② ③ 4 5 6
BM #2 ① ② ③ 4 5 6   BM #4 ① ② ③ 4 5 6

BM Notes ▸ _____

🩺 **Do you need to call your doctor?** | YES | | NO |

15

◯▷ **Breakfast** ▙_____

_____

◯ **Snack** ▙_____

_____

▢ **Lunch** ▙_____

_____

◎ **Snack** ▙_____

_____

🐑 **Dinner** ▙_____

_____

◫─◫ **Exercise** ▙_____ ⏱ **Time Spent Exercising** ▙_____

✓ **What is one good thing that happened today?**

▙_____

⤴ **What can you do to improve tomorrow?**

▙_____

▦ **Personal Journal / Notes** (write something about your day or personal thoughts)

▙_____

_____

_____

_____

_____

_____

_____

Tip: In addition to brushing your teeth, use a mouthwash. Doing something as simple as this can help you to avoid infections.

DAY 009

📅 **Date** _____

🌡️ **Temperature** _____   ⚖️ **Weight** _____

💊 **Medications Taken Today**

1 _____   2 _____   3 _____

Pain (Circle most painful moment)

0 — 1 — 2 — 3 — 4 — 5 — 6 — 7 — 8 — 9 — 10

GOOD   BAD

Types of Pain (circle all that apply)

DULL   **THROBBING**   **SHARP**   **CRAMPING**

How long did the pain last? (circle the longest time)

0 1 2 3 4 5 6 7 8 9 10 11 12 13 14 15 16 17 18 19 20 More +

Minutes

How many times have you experienced pain today? _____

⚡ **Sickness Symptoms** (cough, sweats, feel cold, loss of appetite)

_____

Bowel Movements (bowel movement scale: 1 = Loose // 6 = Hard)

BM #1 ❶ ❷ ❸ 4 5 6   BM #3 ❶ ❷ ❸ 4 5 6

BM #2 ❶ ❷ ❸ ❹ 5 6   BM #4 ❶ ❷ ❸ 4 5 6

BM Notes _____

🩺 **Do you need to call your doctor?**   YES   NO

17

◯ **Breakfast** _____
_____

◯ **Snack** _____
_____

◻ **Lunch** _____
_____

◯ **Snack** _____
_____

◯ **Dinner** _____
_____

◻ **Exercise** _____   ◯ **Time Spent Exercising** _____

✔ **What is one good thing that happened today?**

_____

◀ **What can you do to improve tomorrow?**

_____

▤ **Personal Journal / Notes** (write something about your day or personal thoughts)

_____
_____
_____
_____
_____
_____
_____

Famous People with IBD: John F. Kennedy, the 35th president of the United States, also suffered from adrenal deficiency, osteoporosis, and multiple infections throughout his presidency.

DAY 010

Date _____

Temperature _____   **Weight** _____

Medications Taken Today

1 _____   2 _____   3 _____

Pain (Circle most painful moment)

0 — 1 — 2 — 3 — 4 — 5 — 6 — 7 — 8 — 9 — (10)

GOOD   BAD

Types of Pain (circle all that apply)

DULL | THROBBING | SHARP | CRAMPING

How long did the pain last? (circle the longest time)

0 1 2 3 4 5 6 7 8 9 10 11 12 13 14 15 16 17 18 19 20 [More +]

Minutes

How many times have you experienced pain today? _____

Sickness Symptoms (cough, sweats, feel cold, loss of appetite)

_____

Bowel Movements (bowel movement scale: 1 = Loose // 6 = Hard)

BM #1 ① ② ③ 4 5 6   BM #3 ① ② ③ 4 5 6

BM #2 ① ② ③ 4 5 6   BM #4 ① ② ③ 4 5 6

BM Notes _____

Do you need to call your doctor?   YES   NO

19

Breakfast _____

_____

Snack _____

_____

Lunch _____

_____

Snack _____

_____

Dinner _____

_____

Exercise _____ Time Spent Exercising _____

What is one good thing that happened today?

_____

What can you do to improve tomorrow?

_____

Personal Journal / Notes (write something about your day or personal thoughts)

_____

_____

_____

_____

_____

_____

_____

Tip: Use the "Questions for Doctor_____" portion of this journal to keep a set of questions for your doctor for every visit. The more you ask, the more you will know and the better off you will be.

Date _____

DAY 011

Temperature _____   👁 Weight _____

Medications Taken Today

1 _____   2 _____   3 _____

Pain (Circle most painful moment)

0 — 1 — 2 — 3 — 4 — 5 — 6 — 7 — 8 — 9 — (10)

GOOD   BAD

Types of Pain (circle all that apply)

DULL | THROBBING | SHARP | CRAMPING

How long did the pain last? (circle the longest time)

0 1 2 3 4 5 6 7 8 9 10 11 12 13 14 15 16 17 18 19 20 [More +]

Minutes

How many times have you experienced pain today? _____

⚡ Sickness Symptoms (cough, sweats, feel cold, loss of appetite)

Bowel Movements (bowel movement scale: 1 = Loose // 6 = Hard)

BM #1 ① ② ③ 4 5 6   BM #3 ① ② ③ 4 5 6
BM #2 ① ② ③ 4 5 6   BM #4 ① ② ③ 4 5 6

BM Notes _____

Do you need to call your doctor?   YES   NO

◯ **Breakfast** _____

◉ **Snack** _____

▢ **Lunch** _____

◉ **Snack** _____

🍗 **Dinner** _____

▢-▢ **Exercise** _____ ⏱ **Time Spent Exercising** _____

✓ **What is one good thing that happened today?**

_____

📌 **What can you do to improve tomorrow?**

_____

📋 **Personal Journal / Notes** (write something about your day or personal thoughts)

_____

_____

_____

_____

_____

_____

_____

Did you know?: White rice is a great staple and fallback if you are experiencing symptoms. It is easy to digest and contains calories, which can help during flares.

📅 **Date** _____

DAY 012

🌡 **Temperature** _____   ⊙ **Weight** _____

💊 **Medications Taken Today**

1 _____   2 _____   3 _____

Pain (Circle most painful moment)

0 — 1 — 2 — 3 — 4 — 5 — 6 — 7 — 8 — 9 — 10

GOOD   BAD

Types of Pain (circle all that apply)

| DULL | THROBBING | SHARP | CRAMPING |

How long did the pain last? (circle the longest time)

0 1 2 3 4 5 6 7 8 9 10 11 12 13 14 15 16 17 18 19 20 [More +]

Minutes

How many times have you experienced pain today? ▶ _____

⚡ **Sickness Symptoms** (cough, sweats, feel cold, loss of appetite)

⚗ **Bowel Movements** (bowel movement scale: 1 = Loose // 6 = Hard)

BM #1   ① ② ③ ④ ⑤ ⑥   BM #3   ① ② ③ ④ ⑤ ⑥

BM #2   ① ② ③ ④ ⑤ ⑥   BM #4   ① ② ③ ④ ⑤ ⑥

BM Notes ▶ _____

🩺 **Do you need to call your doctor?**   [YES]   [NO]

23

◯▷ **Breakfast** _____

◉ **Snack** _____

▢ **Lunch** _____

◉ **Snack** _____

🐔 **Dinner** _____

▣ **Exercise** _____ ⏱ **Time Spent Exercising** _____

✅ **What is one good thing that happened today?**

_____

➕ **What can you do to improve tomorrow?**

_____

▦ **Personal Journal / Notes** (write something about your day or personal thoughts)

_____

_____

_____

_____

_____

_____

Famous People with IBD: Cynthia McFadden, news correspondent for ABC News and co-anchor of Primetime and Nightline.

DAY 013

📅 **Date** _____

🌡️ **Temperature** _____ ⚖️ **Weight** _____

💊 **Medications Taken Today**

1 _____ 2 _____ 3 _____

Pain (Circle most painful moment)

0 1 2 3 4 5 6 7 8 9 10
GOOD   BAD

Types of Pain (circle all that apply)

| DULL | THROBBING | SHARP | CRAMPING |

How long did the pain last? (circle the longest time)

0 1 2 3 4 5 6 7 8 9 10 11 12 13 14 15 16 17 18 19 20 More +
Minutes

How many times have you experienced pain today? _____

⚡ **Sickness Symptoms** (cough, sweats, feel cold, loss of appetite)

_____

🚽 **Bowel Movements** (bowel movement scale: 1 = Loose // 6 = Hard)

BM #1 1 2 3 4 5 6   BM #3 1 2 3 4 5 6

BM #2 1 2 3 4 5 6   BM #4 1 2 3 4 5 6

BM Notes _____

🩺 **Do you need to call your doctor?**   YES   NO

25

◯▷ **Breakfast** _____
_____

◯ **Snack** _____
_____

▢ **Lunch** _____
_____

◯ **Snack** _____
_____

Dinner _____
_____

Exercise _____ ⏱ **Time Spent Exercising** _____

✅ **What is one good thing that happened today?**
_____

📌 **What can you do to improve tomorrow?**
_____

📋 **Personal Journal / Notes** (write something about your day or personal thoughts)
_____
_____
_____
_____
_____
_____

> **Tip:** Avoid food with large indigestible fibers. If it looks like it won't digest, it probably won't. Some examples include corn, nuts, raw veggies, and raw fruits with skins or thick fibers. The good news is that many raw veggies and fruits can be cooked to make them easily digestible.

Date _____

DAY 014

Temperature _____ **Weight** _____

Medications Taken Today

1 _____ 2 _____ 3 _____

Pain (Circle most painful moment)

0 1 2 3 4 5 6 7 8 9 10
GOOD   BAD

Types of Pain (circle all that apply)

DULL | THROBBING | SHARP | CRAMPING

How long did the pain last? (circle the longest time)

0 1 2 3 4 5 6 7 8 9 10 11 12 13 14 15 16 17 18 19 20 | More +
Minutes

How many times have you experienced pain today? _____

Sickness Symptoms (cough, sweats, feel cold, loss of appetite)

_____

Bowel Movements (bowel movement scale: 1 = Loose // 6 = Hard)

BM #1 1 2 3 4 5 6   BM #3 1 2 3 4 5 6
BM #2 1 2 3 4 5 6   BM #4 1 2 3 4 5 6

BM Notes _____

Do you need to call your doctor?   YES   NO

○▷ **Breakfast** ▸_____

_____

◉ **Snack** ▸_____

_____

▢ **Lunch** ▸_____

_____

◉ **Snack** ▸_____

_____

🎧 **Dinner** ▸_____

_____

▢-▢ **Exercise** ▸_____ 🕐 **Time Spent Exercising** ▸_____

✅ **What is one good thing that happened today?**

▸_____

📌 **What can you do to improve tomorrow?**

▸_____

📋 **Personal Journal / Notes** (write something about your day or personal thoughts)

▸_____

_____

_____

_____

_____

_____

📅 **Date** _____

DAY 015

🌡 **Temperature** _____   ⬜ **Weight** _____

💊 **Medications Taken Today**

1 _____   2 _____   3 _____

Pain (Circle most painful moment)

0 — 1 — 2 — 3 — 4 — 5 — 6 — 7 — 8 — 9 — 10

GOOD   BAD

Types of Pain (circle all that apply)

DULL | **THROBBING** | **SHARP** | **CRAMPING**

How long did the pain last? (circle the longest time)

0 1 2 3 4 5 6 7 8 9 10 11 12 13 14 15 16 17 18 19 20 [More +]

Minutes

How many times have you experienced pain today? _____

⚡ **Sickness Symptoms** (cough, sweats, feel cold, loss of appetite)

_____

Bowel Movements (bowel movement scale: 1 = Loose // 6 = Hard)

BM #1 ❶ ❷ ❸ ❹ ❺ ❻   BM #3 ❶ ❷ ❸ ❹ ❺ ❻

BM #2 ❶ ❷ ❸ ❹ ❺ ❻   BM #4 ❶ ❷ ❸ ❹ ❺ ❻

BM Notes _____

🩺 **Do you need to call your doctor?**   YES   NO

◯▷ **Breakfast** _____

◯ **Snack** _____

▢ **Lunch** _____

◯ **Snack** _____

🍗 **Dinner** _____

◻◻ **Exercise** _____ 🕐 **Time Spent Exercising** _____

✓ **What is one good thing that happened today?**

_____

+1 **What can you do to improve tomorrow?**

_____

▤ **Personal Journal / Notes** (write something about your day or personal thoughts)

_____

_____

_____

_____

_____

_____

_____

Tip: Try Boost or Ensure as a simple between-meal snack. It is pumped full of nutrients, minerals, and protein.

DAY 016

📅 **Date** _____

🌡 **Temperature** _____   ⚖ **Weight** _____

💊 **Medications Taken Today**

1 _____   2 _____   3 _____

Pain (Circle most painful moment)

0 — 1 — 2 — 3 — 4 — 5 — 6 — 7 — 8 — 9 — **10**
GOOD   BAD

Types of Pain (circle all that apply)

DULL | **THROBBING** | **SHARP** | **CRAMPING**

How long did the pain last? (circle the longest time)

0 1 2 3 4 5 6 7 8 9 10 11 12 13 14 15 16 17 18 19 20 [More +]
Minutes

How many times have you experienced pain today? _____

⚡ **Sickness Symptoms** (cough, sweats, feel cold, loss of appetite)

_____

Bowel Movements (bowel movement scale: 1 = Loose // 6 = Hard)

BM #1 ① ② ③ 4 5 6   BM #3 ① ② ③ 4 5 6

BM #2 ① ② ③ 4 5 6   BM #4 ① ② ③ 4 5 6

BM Notes _____

🩺 **Do you need to call your doctor?**   YES   NO

○D **Breakfast** ▸_____
_____

◉ **Snack** ▸_____
_____

▢ **Lunch** ▸_____
_____

◉ **Snack** ▸_____
_____

🎧 **Dinner** ▸_____
_____

□-□ **Exercise** ▸_____ ⏱ **Time Spent Exercising** ▸_____

✅ **What is one good thing that happened today?**

▸_____

📌 **What can you do to improve tomorrow?**

▸_____

📋 **Personal Journal / Notes** (write something about your day or personal thoughts)

▸_____
_____
_____
_____
_____
_____
_____

Famous People with IBD: Kevin Dineen, former NHL player and current hockey coach of the Florida Panthers.

DAY 017

📅 **Date** _____

🌡 **Temperature** _____   👁 **Weight** _____

💊 **Medications Taken Today**

1 _____   2 _____   3 _____

Pain (Circle most painful moment)

0 — 1 — 2 — 3 — 4 — 5 — 6 — 7 — 8 — 9 — **10**
GOOD   BAD

Types of Pain (circle all that apply)

| DULL | THROBBING | SHARP | CRAMPING |

How long did the pain last? (circle the longest time)

0 1 2 3 4 5 6 7 8 9 10 11 12 13 14 15 16 17 18 19 20   [More +]
Minutes

How many times have you experienced pain today? _____

⚡ **Sickness Symptoms** (cough, sweats, feel cold, loss of appetite)

_____

🚽 **Bowel Movements** (bowel movement scale: 1 = Loose // 6 = Hard)

BM #1 ① ② ③ 4 5 6   BM #3 ① ② ③ 4 5 6
BM #2 ① ② ③ 4 5 6   BM #4 ① ② ③ 4 5 6

BM Notes _____

🩺 **Do you need to call your doctor?**   YES   NO

◯⊃ **Breakfast** ▸_____

_____

◉ **Snack** ▸_____

_____

⬜ **Lunch** ▸_____

_____

◉ **Snack** ▸_____

_____

🍗 **Dinner** ▸_____

_____

◻—◻ **Exercise** ▸_____ ⏱ **Time Spent Exercising** ▸_____

✅ **What is one good thing that happened today?**

▸_____

📌 **What can you do to improve tomorrow?**

▸_____

📋 **Personal Journal / Notes** (write something about your day or personal thoughts)

▸_____

_____

_____

_____

_____

_____

_____

Tip: Maintain a normal sleep schedule. Maintaining a simple schedule helps you to know when you may be experiencing an increase in symptoms and may help you to head off a flare.

Date _____

DAY 018

Temperature _____   **Weight** _____

Medications Taken Today

1 _____   2 _____   3 _____

Pain (Circle most painful moment)

0 1 2 3 4 5 6 7 8 9 10

GOOD   BAD

Types of Pain (circle all that apply)

DULL | THROBBING | SHARP | CRAMPING

How long did the pain last? (circle the longest time)

0 1 2 3 4 5 6 7 8 9 10 11 12 13 14 15 16 17 18 19 20 [More +]

Minutes

How many times have you experienced pain today? _____

Sickness Symptoms (cough, sweats, feel cold, loss of appetite)

Bowel Movements (bowel movement scale: 1 = Loose // 6 = Hard)

BM #1 1 2 3 4 5 6   BM #3 1 2 3 4 5 6

BM #2 1 2 3 4 5 6   BM #4 1 2 3 4 5 6

BM Notes _____

Do you need to call your doctor?   YES   NO

35

◯⃝ **Breakfast** ▸_____
_____

◉ **Snack** ▸_____
_____

▢ **Lunch** ▸_____
_____

◉ **Snack** ▸_____
_____

🐷 **Dinner** ▸_____
_____

⊶ **Exercise** ▸_____   ⏱ **Time Spent Exercising** ▸_____

✅ **What is one good thing that happened today?**

▸_____

📌 **What can you do to improve tomorrow?**

▸_____

▤ **Personal Journal / Notes** (write something about your day or personal thoughts)

▸_____
_____
_____
_____
_____
_____

⊕ Tip: Stay intimate. Don't shy away from intimacy because of symptoms: Let your partner know what feels good, such as kissing, hugging or just being together.

📅 **Date** ⬊_____

DAY 019

🌡 **Temperature** ⬊_____ 👁 **Weight** ⬊_____

💊 **Medications Taken Today**

1 ⬊_____ 2 ⬊_____ 3 ⬊_____

🩹 **Pain** (Circle most painful moment)

0 — 1 — 2 — 3 — 4 — 5 — 6 — 7 — 8 — 9 — **10**
GOOD   BAD

Types of Pain (circle all that apply)

| DULL | THROBBING | SHARP | CRAMPING |

How long did the pain last? (circle the longest time)

0 1 2 3 4 5 6 7 8 9 10 11 12 13 14 15 16 17 18 19 20 [More +]
Minutes

How many times have you experienced pain today? ⬊_____

⚡ **Sickness Symptoms** (cough, sweats, feel cold, loss of appetite)

_____

🏺 **Bowel Movements** (bowel movement scale: 1 = Loose // 6 = Hard)

BM #1 ❶ ❷ 3 4 5 6   BM #3 ❶ ❷ ❸ 4 5 6

BM #2 ❶ ❷ ❸ ❹ 5 6   BM #4 ❶ ❷ 3 4 5 6

BM Notes ⬊_____

🩺 **Do you need to call your doctor?**   YES   NO

◯⊃ **Breakfast** ▶_____

_____

◉ **Snack** ▶_____

_____

▢ **Lunch** ▶_____

_____

◉ **Snack** ▶_____

_____

♔ **Dinner** ▶_____

_____

⊡-O **Exercise** ▶_____   ⏱ **Time Spent Exercising** ▶_____

✔ **What is one good thing that happened today?**

▶_____

📑 **What can you do to improve tomorrow?**

▶_____

▤ **Personal Journal / Notes** (write something about your day or personal thoughts)

▶_____

_____

_____

_____

_____

_____

_____

Tip: Ask your doctor to write down all instructions and details from your visit. Keeping these in chronological order can help future doctors' overview your treatment and past.

📅 **Date** _____

DAY 020

🌡 **Temperature** _____   ⚖ **Weight** _____

💊 **Medications Taken Today**

1 _____   2 _____   3 _____

Pain (Circle most painful moment)

0 — 1 — 2 — 3 — 4 — 5 — 6 — 7 — 8 — 9 — (10)
GOOD   BAD

Types of Pain (circle all that apply)

| DULL | THROBBING | SHARP | CRAMPING |

How long did the pain last? (circle the longest time)

0 1 2 3 4 5 6 7 8 9 10 11 12 13 14 15 16 17 18 19 20 [More +]
Minutes

How many times have you experienced pain today? _____

⚡ **Sickness Symptoms** (cough, sweats, feel cold, loss of appetite)

_____

Bowel Movements (bowel movement scale: 1 = Loose // 6 = Hard)

BM #1 ① ② ③ 4 5 6   BM #3 ① ② ③ 4 5 6

BM #2 ① ② ③ 4 5 6   BM #4 ① ② ③ 4 5 6

BM Notes _____

🩺 **Do you need to call your doctor?** | YES | | NO |

39

◯ **Breakfast** _____

_____

◯ **Snack** _____

_____

◻ **Lunch** _____

_____

◯ **Snack** _____

_____

◯ **Dinner** _____

_____

Exercise _____ ◯ **Time Spent Exercising** _____

✓ **What is one good thing that happened today?**

_____

What can you do to improve tomorrow?

_____

▤ **Personal Journal / Notes** (write something about your day or personal thoughts)

_____

_____

_____

_____

_____

_____

_____

Did you know?: You don't have to avoid all fruits! Bananas, papaya, cantaloupe, and mango are all easily digestible fruits that are rich in vitamins and minerals, many of which can aid in the digestion of proteins.

DAY 021

Date _____

Temperature _____   **Weight** _____

Medications Taken Today

1 _____   2 _____   3 _____

Pain (Circle most painful moment)

0 — 1 — 2 — 3 — 4 — 5 — 6 — 7 — 8 — 9 — 10
GOOD   BAD

Types of Pain (circle all that apply)

DULL | THROBBING | SHARP | CRAMPING

How long did the pain last? (circle the longest time)

0 1 2 3 4 5 6 7 8 9 10 11 12 13 14 15 16 17 18 19 20 [More +]
Minutes

How many times have you experienced pain today? _____

Sickness Symptoms (cough, sweats, feel cold, loss of appetite)

_____

Bowel Movements (bowel movement scale: 1 = Loose // 6 = Hard)

BM #1 1 2 3 4 5 6   BM #3 1 2 3 4 5 6
BM #2 1 2 3 4 5 6   BM #4 1 2 3 4 5 6

BM Notes _____

Do you need to call your doctor?   YES   NO

Breakfast _____

_____

Snack _____

_____

Lunch _____

_____

Snack _____

_____

Dinner _____

_____

Exercise _____ Time Spent Exercising _____

What is one good thing that happened today?

_____

What can you do to improve tomorrow?

_____

Personal Journal / Notes (write something about your day or personal thoughts)

_____

_____

_____

_____

_____

_____

Did you know?: Most doctors recommend that you only use Tylenol, or a similar generic, as an over-the-counter medicine to manage mild pain. This is because it is less harsh on your system.

DAY 022

Date ________________

Temperature ________ **Weight** ________

Medications Taken Today

1 ________ 2 ________ 3 ________

Pain (Circle most painful moment)

0 1 2 3 4 5 6 7 8 9 10

GOOD BAD

Types of Pain (circle all that apply)

DULL | THROBBING | SHARP | CRAMPING

How long did the pain last? (circle the longest time)

0 1 2 3 4 5 6 7 8 9 10 11 12 13 14 15 16 17 18 19 20 More +

Minutes

How many times have you experienced pain today? ________

Sickness Symptoms (cough, sweats, feel cold, loss of appetite)

Bowel Movements (bowel movement scale: 1 = Loose // 6 = Hard)

BM #1 1 2 3 4 5 6 **BM #3** 1 2 3 4 5 6

BM #2 1 2 3 4 5 6 **BM #4** 1 2 3 4 5 6

BM Notes ________________

Do you need to call your doctor? YES NO

◯▷ **Breakfast** _____

_____

◯ **Snack** _____

_____

▢ **Lunch** _____

_____

◯ **Snack** _____

_____

Dinner _____

_____

☐━☐ **Exercise** _____   ◷ **Time Spent Exercising** _____

✓ **What is one good thing that happened today?**

_____

What can you do to improve tomorrow?

_____

▤ **Personal Journal / Notes** (write something about your day or personal thoughts)

_____

_____

_____

_____

_____

_____

_____

> **Tip:** Schedule something in your week to look forward to, whether it be movies with a friend or a public outing. Use this as motivational force if your week hasn't gone quite as planned.

Date _____

DAY 023

Temperature _____   **Weight** _____

Medications Taken Today

1 _____   2 _____   3 _____

Pain (Circle most painful moment)

0 — 1 — 2 — 3 — 4 — 5 — 6 — 7 — 8 — 9 — 10
GOOD   BAD

Types of Pain (circle all that apply)

| DULL | THROBBING | SHARP | CRAMPING |

How long did the pain last? (circle the longest time)

0 1 2 3 4 5 6 7 8 9 10 11 12 13 14 15 16 17 18 19 20 [More +]
Minutes

How many times have you experienced pain today? _____

Sickness Symptoms (cough, sweats, feel cold, loss of appetite)

_____

Bowel Movements (bowel movement scale: 1 = Loose // 6 = Hard)

BM #1 ❶ ❷ ③ 4 5 6   BM #3 ❶ ❷ ③ 4 5 6

BM #2 ❶ ❷ ③ 4 5 6   BM #4 ❶ ❷ ③ 4 5 6

BM Notes _____

Do you need to call your doctor?   YES   NO

45

◯▷ **Breakfast** ▸_____

_____

◉ **Snack** ▸_____

_____

▢ **Lunch** ▸_____

_____

◉ **Snack** ▸_____

_____

🍄 **Dinner** ▸_____

_____

〇-〇 **Exercise** ▸_____ ⏱ **Time Spent Exercising** ▸_____

✓ **What is one good thing that happened today?**

▸_____

⚑ **What can you do to improve tomorrow?**

▸_____

▤ **Personal Journal / Notes** (write something about your day or personal thoughts)

▸_____

_____

_____

_____

_____

_____

_____

✚ Famous People with IBD: Anastacia, a widely popular American singer/songwriter.

📅 **Date** _____

DAY 024

🌡️ **Temperature** _____ 👁️ **Weight** _____

💊 **Medications Taken Today**

1 _____ 2 _____ 3 _____

Pain (Circle most painful moment)

0 1 2 3 4 5 6 7 8 9 10
GOOD   BAD

Types of Pain (circle all that apply)

| DULL | THROBBING | SHARP | CRAMPING |

How long did the pain last? (circle the longest time)

0 1 2 3 4 5 6 7 8 9 10 11 12 13 14 15 16 17 18 19 20 [More +]
Minutes

How many times have you experienced pain today? _____

⚡ **Sickness Symptoms** (cough, sweats, feel cold, loss of appetite)

_____

🚽 **Bowel Movements** (bowel movement scale: 1 = Loose // 6 = Hard)

BM #1 ① ② ③ ④ ⑤ ⑥   BM #3 ① ② ③ ④ ⑤ ⑥
BM #2 ① ② ③ ④ ⑤ ⑥   BM #4 ① ② ③ ④ ⑤ ⑥

BM Notes _____

🩺 **Do you need to call your doctor?** YES   NO

47

◯▷ **Breakfast** _____

_____

◯ **Snack** _____

_____

▢ **Lunch** _____

_____

◯ **Snack** _____

_____

🎧 **Dinner** _____

_____

⌿ **Exercise** _____ ⏱ **Time Spent Exercising** _____

✔ **What is one good thing that happened today?**

_____

📌 **What can you do to improve tomorrow?**

_____

📄 **Personal Journal / Notes** (write something about your day or personal thoughts)

_____

_____

_____

_____

_____

_____

_____

Did you know?: Taking a calcium tablet along with your morning vitamins is recommended by many doctors. This is because some medications, specifically corticosteroids, can increase risk for osteoporosis, and in specific cases it may help to reduce chances of kidney stones.

📅 **Date** _____

DAY 025

🌡 **Temperature** _____   ⚖ **Weight** _____

💊 **Medications Taken Today**

1 _____   2 _____   3 _____

Pain (Circle most painful moment)

0 1 2 3 4 5 6 7 8 9 10
GOOD   BAD

Types of Pain (circle all that apply)

| DULL | THROBBING | SHARP | CRAMPING |

How long did the pain last? (circle the longest time)

0 1 2 3 4 5 6 7 8 9 10 11 12 13 14 15 16 17 18 19 20 More +
Minutes

How many times have you experienced pain today? _____

⚡ **Sickness Symptoms** (cough, sweats, feel cold, loss of appetite)

_____

Bowel Movements (bowel movement scale: 1 = Loose // 6 = Hard)

BM #1 1 2 3 4 5 6   BM #3 1 2 3 4 5 6
BM #2 1 2 3 4 5 6   BM #4 1 2 3 4 5 6

BM Notes _____

🩺 **Do you need to call your doctor?**   YES   NO

◯▷ **Breakfast** ▶_____

_____

◯ **Snack** ▶_____

_____

▢ **Lunch** ▶_____

_____

◯ **Snack** ▶_____

_____

🎧 **Dinner** ▶_____

_____

▢▢ **Exercise** ▶_____ ◯ **Time Spent Exercising** ▶_____

✅ **What is one good thing that happened today?**

▶_____

📌 **What can you do to improve tomorrow?**

▶_____

📄 **Personal Journal / Notes** (write something about your day or personal thoughts)

▶_____

_____

_____

_____

_____

_____

_____

Did you know?: Stress can affect the body hours after the stressful situation has passed. Muscles can remain flexed and taut, causing chain reactions throughout your body, including your gut. Try taking a walk or exercising directly after a stressful event to head off any symptoms.

Date _____

DAY 026

Temperature _____ _____   **Weight** _____ _____

Medications Taken Today

1 _____ 2 _____ 3 _____

Pain (Circle most painful moment)

0   1   2   3   4   5   6   7   8   9   10
GOOD   BAD

Types of Pain (circle all that apply)

| DULL | THROBBING | SHARP | CRAMPING |

How long did the pain last? (circle the longest time)

0 1 2 3 4 5 6 7 8 9 10 11 12 13 14 15 16 17 18 19 20 [More +]

Minutes

How many times have you experienced pain today? _____

Sickness Symptoms (cough, sweats, feel cold, loss of appetite)

_____

Bowel Movements (bowel movement scale: 1 = Loose // 6 = Hard)

BM #1   ❶ ❷ ❸ 4 5 6   BM #3   ❶ ❷ ❸ 4 5 6

BM #2   ❶ ❷ ❸ 4 5 6   BM #4   ❶ ❷ ❸ 4 5 6

BM Notes _____

Do you need to call your doctor?   YES   NO

○○ **Breakfast** _____

_____

◎ **Snack** _____

_____

▢ **Lunch** _____

_____

◎ **Snack** _____

_____

🐑 **Dinner** _____

_____

○─○ **Exercise** _____ ⊘ **Time Spent Exercising** _____

✅ **What is one good thing that happened today?**

_____

⚑ **What can you do to improve tomorrow?**

_____

▤ **Personal Journal / Notes** (write something about your day or personal thoughts)

_____

_____

_____

_____

_____

_____

Did You Know?: You are at high risk of dehydration during a flare. Drink water as much as possible to reduce symptoms and increase your body's ability to recover.

📅 **Date** _____

DAY 027

🌡 **Temperature** _____   ⊙ **Weight** _____

💊 **Medications Taken Today**

1 _____   2 _____   3 _____

Pain (Circle most painful moment)

0 — 1 — 2 — 3 — 4 — 5 — 6 — 7 — 8 — 9 — 10
GOOD   BAD

Types of Pain (circle all that apply)

| DULL | THROBBING | SHARP | CRAMPING |

How long did the pain last? (circle the longest time)

0 1 2 3 4 5 6 7 8 9 10 11 12 13 14 15 16 17 18 19 20 [More +]

Minutes

How many times have you experienced pain today? _____

⚡ **Sickness Symptoms** (cough, sweats, feel cold, loss of appetite)

_____

Bowel Movements (bowel movement scale: 1 = Loose // 6 = Hard)

BM #1 ① ② ③ ④ ⑤ ⑥   BM #3 ① ② ③ ④ ⑤ ⑥

BM #2 ① ② ③ ④ ⑤ ⑥   BM #4 ① ② ③ ④ ⑤ ⑥

BM Notes _____

🩺 **Do you need to call your doctor?**   YES   NO

◯ **Breakfast** _____

_____

◯ **Snack** _____

_____

▢ **Lunch** _____

_____

◯ **Snack** _____

_____

🐑 **Dinner** _____

_____

□-□ **Exercise** _____ 🕐 **Time Spent Exercising** _____

✅ **What is one good thing that happened today?**

_____

📌 **What can you do to improve tomorrow?**

_____

📋 **Personal Journal / Notes** (write something about your day or personal thoughts)

_____

_____

_____

_____

_____

_____

_____

📅 **Date** _____

DAY 028

🌡️ **Temperature** _____ 👁️ **Weight** _____

💊 **Medications Taken Today**

1 _____ 2 _____ 3 _____

Pain (Circle most painful moment)

0 1 2 3 4 5 6 7 8 9 10

GOOD   BAD

Types of Pain (circle all that apply)

DULL | THROBBING | SHARP | CRAMPING

How long did the pain last? (circle the longest time)

0 1 2 3 4 5 6 7 8 9 10 11 12 13 14 15 16 17 18 19 20 | More +

Minutes

How many times have you experienced pain today? _____

⚡ **Sickness Symptoms** (cough, sweats, feel cold, loss of appetite)

_____

Bowel Movements (bowel movement scale: 1 = Loose // 6 = Hard)

BM #1 ① ② ③ ④ ⑤ ⑥   BM #3 ① ② ③ ④ ⑤ ⑥

BM #2 ① ② ③ ④ ⑤ ⑥   BM #4 ① ② ③ ④ ⑤ ⑥

BM Notes _____

🩺 **Do you need to call your doctor?** YES NO

Breakfast _____
_____

 Snack _____
_____

 Lunch _____
_____

 Snack _____
_____

 Dinner _____
_____

 Exercise _____   Time Spent Exercising _____

 What is one good thing that happened today?

_____

 What can you do to improve tomorrow?

_____

 Personal Journal / Notes (write something about your day or personal thoughts)

_____
_____
_____
_____
_____
_____
_____

31 Date _____

DAY 029

Temperature _____ **Weight** _____

Medications Taken Today

1 _____ 2 _____ 3 _____

Pain (Circle most painful moment)

⓪ ① ② ③ ④ ⑤ ⑥ ⑦ ⑧ ⑨ **⑩**

GOOD   BAD

Types of Pain (circle all that apply)

DULL | **THROBBING** | **SHARP** | **CRAMPING**

How long did the pain last? (circle the longest time)

0 1 2 3 4 5 6 7 8 9 10 11 12 13 14 15 16 17 18 19 20 | More + |

Minutes

How many times have you experienced pain today? _____

Sickness Symptoms (cough, sweats, feel cold, loss of appetite)

_____

Bowel Movements (bowel movement scale: 1 = Loose // 6 = Hard)

BM #1 ❶ ❷ ❸ 4 5 6   BM #3 ❶ ❷ ❸ 4 5 6

BM #2 ❶ ❷ ❸ 4 5 6   BM #4 ❶ ❷ ❸ 4 5 6

BM Notes _____

Do you need to call your doctor?   [YES]   [NO]

◯◗ **Breakfast** ▸_____

◯ **Snack** ▸_____

◻ **Lunch** ▸_____

◯ **Snack** ▸_____

◯◯ **Dinner** ▸_____

▭▭ **Exercise** ▸_____ ◷ **Time Spent Exercising** ▸_____

✔ **What is one good thing that happened today?**

▸_____

✦1 **What can you do to improve tomorrow?**

▸_____

▤ **Personal Journal / Notes** (write something about your day or personal thoughts)

▸_____

_____

_____

_____

_____

_____

📅 **Date** ◣_____

DAY 030

🌡️ **Temperature** ◣_____   👁️ **Weight** ◣_____

💊 **Medications Taken Today**

1 ◣_____   2 ◣_____   3 ◣_____

Pain (Circle most painful moment)

0 — 1 — 2 — 3 — 4 — 5 — 6 — 7 — 8 — 9 — 10
GOOD   BAD

Types of Pain (circle all that apply)

| DULL | THROBBING | SHARP | CRAMPING |

How long did the pain last? (circle the longest time)

0 1 2 3 4 5 6 7 8 9 10 11 12 13 14 15 16 17 18 19 20 [More +]
Minutes

How many times have you experienced pain today? ◣

⚡ **Sickness Symptoms** (cough, sweats, feel cold, loss of appetite)

_____

🫖 **Bowel Movements** (bowel movement scale: 1 = Loose // 6 = Hard)

BM #1 ① ② ③ ④ ⑤ ⑥   BM #3 ① ② ③ ④ ⑤ ⑥
BM #2 ① ② ③ ④ ⑤ ⑥   BM #4 ① ② ③ ④ ⑤ ⑥

BM Notes ◣_____

🩺 **Do you need to call your doctor?**   YES   NO

◯ Breakfast _____

◯ Snack _____

◻ Lunch _____

◯ Snack _____

◯ Dinner _____

◻─◻ Exercise _____ ◯ Time Spent Exercising _____

✔ **What is one good thing that happened today?**

_____

•1 **What can you do to improve tomorrow?**

_____

▤ **Personal Journal / Notes** (write something about your day or personal thoughts)

_____

_____

_____

_____

_____

_____

⊕ Tip: Oatmeal, which has soluble fiber, can be a great meal even during a flare. Soluble fiber passes more slowly through the digestive system and absorbs water, which can help with loose stools.

📅 **Date** _____

DAY 031

🌡 **Temperature** _____   👁 **Weight** _____

💊 **Medications Taken Today**

1 _____   2 _____   3 _____

Pain (Circle most painful moment)

0 1 2 3 4 5 6 7 8 9 **10**
GOOD   BAD

Types of Pain (circle all that apply)

DULL | **THROBBING** | **SHARP** | **CRAMPING**

How long did the pain last? (circle the longest time)

0 1 2 3 4 5 6 7 8 9 10 11 12 13 14 15 16 17 18 19 20 [More +]
Minutes

How many times have you experienced pain today? _____

⚡ **Sickness Symptoms** (cough, sweats, feel cold, loss of appetite)

[   ]

Bowel Movements (bowel movement scale: 1 = Loose // 6 = Hard)

BM #1 **1** 2 3 4 5 6   BM #3 **1** 2 3 4 5 6
BM #2 **1** 2 3 4 5 6   BM #4 **1** 2 3 4 5 6

BM Notes _____

🩺 **Do you need to call your doctor?**   YES   NO

61

⊙ **Breakfast** _____
_____

⊙ **Snack** _____
_____

⊡ **Lunch** _____
_____

⊙ **Snack** _____
_____

⊙ **Dinner** _____
_____

⊡ **Exercise** _____ ⏱ **Time Spent Exercising** _____

✔ **What is one good thing that happened today?**
_____

➜ **What can you do to improve tomorrow?**
_____

▤ **Personal Journal / Notes** (write something about your day or personal thoughts)
_____
_____
_____
_____
_____
_____

Tip: Don't forget to ask your doctor about getting your flu shot and pneumonia vaccine. These simple measures can help avoid some nasty downtime.

31 Date _____

DAY 032

Temperature _____   **Weight** _____

Medications Taken Today

1 _____   2 _____   3 _____

Pain (Circle most painful moment)

0   1   2   3   4   5   6   7   8   9   10
GOOD   BAD

Types of Pain (circle all that apply)

DULL | **THROBBING** | **SHARP** | **CRAMPING**

How long did the pain last? (circle the longest time)

0 1 2 3 4 5 6 7 8 9 10 11 12 13 14 15 16 17 18 19 20   More +
Minutes

How many times have you experienced pain today? _____

Sickness Symptoms (cough, sweats, feel cold, loss of appetite)

Bowel Movements (bowel movement scale: 1 = Loose // 6 = Hard)

BM #1   1 2 3 4 5 6   BM #3   1 2 3 4 5 6

BM #2   1 2 3 4 5 6   BM #4   1 2 3 4 5 6

BM Notes _____

Do you need to call your doctor?   YES   NO

○ Breakfast _____

○ Snack _____

○ Lunch _____

○ Snack _____

○ Dinner _____

○○ Exercise _____ ⏱ Time Spent Exercing _____

✓ **What is one good thing that happened today?**

_____

◀ **What can you do to improve tomorrow?**

_____

▤ **Personal Journal / Notes** (write something about your day or personal thoughts)

_____

_____

_____

_____

_____

_____

_____

31 Date _____

DAY 033

Temperature _____   **Weight** _____

Medications Taken Today

1 _____   2 _____   3 _____

Pain (Circle most painful moment)

0 1 2 3 4 5 6 7 8 9 10

GOOD   BAD

Types of Pain (circle all that apply)

DULL | THROBBING | SHARP | CRAMPING

How long did the pain last? (circle the longest time)

0 1 2 3 4 5 6 7 8 9 10 11 12 13 14 15 16 17 18 19 20 [More +]

Minutes

How many times have you experienced pain today? _____

Sickness Symptoms (cough, sweats, feel cold, loss of appetite)

_____

Bowel Movements (bowel movement scale: 1 = Loose // 6 = Hard)

BM #1 1 2 3 4 5 6   BM #3 1 2 3 4 5 6

BM #2 1 2 3 4 5 6   BM #4 1 2 3 4 5 6

BM Notes _____

Do you need to call your doctor?   YES   NO

◯⟩ **Breakfast**

◯ **Snack**

▢ **Lunch**

◯ **Snack**

🍗 **Dinner**

▭▭ **Exercise**   ⏱ **Time Spent Exercising**

✔ **What is one good thing that happened today?**

✦1 **What can you do to improve tomorrow?**

📄 **Personal Journal / Notes** (write something about your day or personal thoughts)

Did you know?: Some IBD patients have claimed that taking Chlorella supplements can help to alleviate gas and decrease toxins in the body. As always, you should consult your doctor before taking any additional supplements or medications.

DAY 034

31 Date _____

Temperature _____ **Weight** _____

Medications Taken Today

1 _____ 2 _____ 3 _____

Pain (Circle most painful moment)

(0) (1) (2) (3) (4) (5) (6) (7) (8) (9) (10)
GOOD   BAD

Types of Pain (circle all that apply)

| DULL | THROBBING | SHARP | CRAMPING |

How long did the pain last? (circle the longest time)

0 1 2 3 4 5 6 7 8 9 10 11 12 13 14 15 16 17 18 19 20 [More +]
Minutes

How many times have you experienced pain today? _____

Sickness Symptoms (cough, sweats, feel cold, loss of appetite)

_____

Bowel Movements (bowel movement scale: 1 = Loose // 6 = Hard)

BM #1 ① ② ③ 4 5 6   BM #3 ① ② ③ 4 5 6
BM #2 ① ② ③ 4 5 6   BM #4 ① ② ③ 4 5 6

BM Notes _____

Do you need to call your doctor?   YES   NO

◯▷ **Breakfast** ▖_____

_____

◯ **Snack** ▖_____

_____

⬜ **Lunch** ▖_____

_____

◯ **Snack** ▖_____

_____

🍄 **Dinner** ▖_____

_____

⊙━⊙ **Exercise** ▖_____ 🕐 **Time Spent Exercising** ▖_____

✅ **What is one good thing that happened today?**

▖_____

📌 **What can you do to improve tomorrow?**

▖_____

📃 **Personal Journal / Notes** (write something about your day or personal thoughts)

▖_____

_____

_____

_____

_____

_____

_____

📅 **Date** ⟍_____

DAY 035

🌡 **Temperature** ⟍_____ 👁 **Weight** ⟍_____

💊 **Medications Taken Today**

1 ⟍_____ 2 ⟍_____ 3 ⟍_____

Pain (Circle most painful moment)

0 — 1 — 2 — 3 — 4 — 5 — 6 — 7 — 8 — 9 — 10
GOOD   BAD

Types of Pain (circle all that apply)

| DULL | THROBBING | SHARP | CRAMPING |

How long did the pain last? (circle the longest time)

0 1 2 3 4 5 6 7 8 9 10 11 12 13 14 15 16 17 18 19 20 [More +]

Minutes

How many times have you experienced pain today? ⟍_____

⚡ **Sickness Symptoms** (cough, sweats, feel cold, loss of appetite)

_____

Bowel Movements (bowel movement scale: 1 = Loose // 6 = Hard)

BM #1 ① ② 3 4 5 6   BM #3 ① ② 3 4 5 6
BM #2 ① ② 3 4 5 6   BM #4 ① ② 3 4 5 6

BM Notes ⟍_____

🩺 **Do you need to call your doctor?** | YES | | NO |

69

○⊃ **Breakfast** ▸_____

_____

◔ **Snack** ▸_____

_____

▢ **Lunch** ▸_____

_____

◎ **Snack** ▸_____

_____

🍗 **Dinner** ▸_____

_____

○–○ **Exercise** ▸_____   ⏱ **Time Spent Exercising** ▸_____

✓ **What is one good thing that happened today?**

▸_____

⚑ **What can you do to improve tomorrow?**

▸_____

▤ **Personal Journal / Notes** (write something about your day or personal thoughts)

▸_____

_____

_____

_____

_____

_____

_____

Tip: When traveling, bring snacks you know will "sit well with" your system; map out bathroom stops and restaurants you know will work well for you.

DAY 036

📅 Date _____

🌡 Temperature _____   ⚖ Weight _____

💊 **Medications Taken Today**

1 _____   2 _____   3 _____

Pain (Circle most painful moment)

0 1 2 3 4 5 6 7 8 9 **10**
GOOD   BAD

Types of Pain (circle all that apply)

DULL | **THROBBING** | **SHARP** | **CRAMPING**

How long did the pain last? (circle the longest time)

0 1 2 3 4 5 6 7 8 9 10 11 12 13 14 15 16 17 18 19 20 [More +]
Minutes

How many times have you experienced pain today? _____

⚡ **Sickness Symptoms** (cough, sweats, feel cold, loss of appetite)

_____

Bowel Movements (bowel movement scale: 1 = Loose // 6 = Hard)

BM #1 ① ② ③ ④ ⑤ ⑥   BM #3 ① ② ③ ④ ⑤ ⑥
BM #2 ① ② ③ ④ ⑤ ⑥   BM #4 ① ② ③ ④ ⑤ ⑥

BM Notes _____

🩺 **Do you need to call your doctor?**   YES   NO

🥚 **Breakfast** _____

_____

⊙ **Snack** _____

_____

🍞 **Lunch** _____

_____

⊙ **Snack** _____

_____

🍗 **Dinner** _____

_____

Exercise _____ ⏱ **Time Spent Exercising** _____

✅ **What is one good thing that happened today?**

_____

📌 **What can you do to improve tomorrow?**

_____

📄 **Personal Journal / Notes** (write something about your day or personal thoughts)

_____

_____

_____

_____

_____

_____

📅 **Date** _____

DAY 037

🌡️ **Temperature** _____   👁️ **Weight** _____

💊 **Medications Taken Today**

1 _____   2 _____   3 _____

🩹 **Pain** (Circle most painful moment)

0　1　2　3　4　5　6　7　8　9　10
GOOD　　　　　　　　　　　　　　　　BAD

Types of Pain (circle all that apply)

DULL | **THROBBING** | **SHARP** | **CRAMPING**

How long did the pain last? (circle the longest time)

0 1 2 3 4 5 6 7 8 9 10 11 12 13 14 15 16 17 18 19 20 [More +]
Minutes

How many times have you experienced pain today? _____

⚡ **Sickness Symptoms** (cough, sweats, feel cold, loss of appetite)

_____

Bowel Movements (bowel movement scale: 1 = Loose // 6 = Hard)

BM #1 ① ② 3 4 5 6   BM #3 ① ② 3 4 5 6
BM #2 ① ② 3 4 5 6   BM #4 ① ② 3 4 5 6

BM Notes _____

🩺 **Do you need to call your doctor?**   [YES]   [NO]

73

🥚 Breakfast _____
_____

🍪 Snack _____
_____

🍞 Lunch _____
_____

🍪 Snack _____
_____

🍗 Dinner _____
_____

🏋 Exercise _____ ⏱ Time Spent Exercising _____

✅ What is one good thing that happened today?

_____

📍 What can you do to improve tomorrow?

_____

📋 Personal Journal / Notes (write something about your day or personal thoughts)

_____
_____
_____
_____
_____
_____
_____
_____

Date ⬛ _____

DAY 038

Temperature ⬛ _____ **Weight** ⬛ _____

Medications Taken Today

1 ⬛ _____ 2 ⬛ _____ 3 ⬛ _____

Pain (Circle most painful moment)

0 1 2 3 4 5 6 7 8 9 10

GOOD   BAD

Types of Pain (circle all that apply)

DULL | THROBBING | SHARP | CRAMPING

How long did the pain last? (circle the longest time)

0 1 2 3 4 5 6 7 8 9 10 11 12 13 14 15 16 17 18 19 20 |More +

Minutes

How many times have you experienced pain today? ⬛ _____

Sickness Symptoms (cough, sweats, feel cold, loss of appetite)

_____

Bowel Movements (bowel movement scale: 1 = Loose // 6 = Hard)

BM #1 **1** **2** 3 4 5 6   BM #3 **1** **2** 3 4 5 6

BM #2 **1** **2** 3 4 5 6   BM #4 **1** **2** 3 4 5 6

BM Notes ⬛ _____

Do you need to call your doctor? YES NO

Breakfast _____

Snack _____

Lunch _____

Snack _____

Dinner _____

Exercise _____ Time Spent Exercising _____

What is one good thing that happened today?
_____

What can you do to improve tomorrow?
_____

Personal Journal / Notes (write something about your day or personal thoughts)
_____
_____
_____
_____
_____
_____
_____

Tip: Try using a blender or blend stick with steamed vegetables such as lentils, butternut squash, parsnips, pumpkin and carrots to make creamy vegetable soups. By blending them, you won't lose as many nutrients as you would boiling and mashing them, and you can still enjoy a healthy nutritious meal.

DAY 039

📅 **Date** _____

🌡 **Temperature** _____   👁 **Weight** _____

💊 **Medications Taken Today**

1 _____   2 _____   3 _____

Pain (Circle most painful moment)

0 — 1 — 2 — 3 — 4 — 5 — 6 — 7 — 8 — 9 — **10**
GOOD   BAD

Types of Pain (circle all that apply)

DULL | **THROBBING** | **SHARP** | **CRAMPING**

How long did the pain last? (circle the longest time)

0 1 2 3 4 5 6 7 8 9 10 11 12 13 14 15 16 17 18 19 20 [More +]
Minutes

How many times have you experienced pain today? _____

⚡ **Sickness Symptoms** (cough, sweats, feel cold, loss of appetite)

_____

Bowel Movements (bowel movement scale: 1 = Loose // 6 = Hard)

BM #1 **1** **2** 3 4 5 6   BM #3 **1** **2** 3 4 5 6

BM #2 **1** **2** 3 **4** 5 6   BM #4 **1** **2** 3 4 5 6

BM Notes _____

🩺 **Do you need to call your doctor?**   YES   NO

◐ **Breakfast** _____

_____

◉ **Snack** _____

_____

▢ **Lunch** _____

_____

◉ **Snack** _____

_____

🐷 **Dinner** _____

_____

🏋 **Exercise** _____ ⏱ **Time Spent Exercising** _____

✔ **What is one good thing that happened today?**

_____

⁺1 **What can you do to improve tomorrow?**

_____

▤ **Personal Journal / Notes** (write something about your day or personal thoughts)

_____

_____

_____

_____

_____

_____

_____

📅 **Date** _____

DAY 040

🌡 **Temperature** _____ 👁 **Weight** _____

💊 **Medications Taken Today**

1 _____ 2 _____ 3 _____

🩹 **Pain** (Circle most painful moment)

0 1 2 3 4 5 6 7 8 9 **10**

GOOD   BAD

Types of Pain (circle all that apply)

| DULL | THROBBING | SHARP | CRAMPING |

How long did the pain last? (circle the longest time)

0 1 2 3 4 5 6 7 8 9 10 11 12 13 14 15 16 17 18 19 20 | More + |

Minutes

How many times have you experienced pain today? _____

⚡ **Sickness Symptoms** (cough, sweats, feel cold, loss of appetite)

_____

🏺 **Bowel Movements** (bowel movement scale: 1 = Loose // 6 = Hard)

BM #1 ① ② 3 4 5 6   BM #3 ① ② 3 4 5 6

BM #2 ① ② 3 4 5 6   BM #4 ① ② 3 4 5 6

BM Notes _____

🩺 **Do you need to call your doctor?** | YES | | NO |

79

◯ **Breakfast** _____

_____

◯ **Snack** _____

_____

◻ **Lunch** _____

_____

◯ **Snack** _____

_____

🍗 **Dinner** _____

_____

◻ **Exercise** _____ 🕐 **Time Spent Exercising** _____

✅ **What is one good thing that happened today?**

_____

➕1 **What can you do to improve tomorrow?**

_____

▦ **Personal Journal / Notes** (write something about your day or personal thoughts)

_____

_____

_____

_____

_____

_____

_____

⊕ Famous People with IBD: Dwight D. Eisenhower, WWII general and 34th president of the United States.

📅 **Date** ▲_____

DAY 041

🌡 **Temperature** ▲_____ ⚖ **Weight** ▲_____

💊 **Medications Taken Today**

1 ▲_____ 2 ▲_____ 3 ▲_____

Pain (Circle most painful moment)

0 — 1 — 2 — 3 — 4 — 5 — 6 — 7 — 8 — 9 — **10**
GOOD   BAD

Types of Pain (circle all that apply)

| DULL | THROBBING | SHARP | CRAMPING |

How long did the pain last? (circle the longest time)

0 1 2 3 4 5 6 7 8 9 10 11 12 13 14 15 16 17 18 19 20 |More +|
Minutes

How many times have you experienced pain today? ▲_____

⚡ **Sickness Symptoms** (cough, sweats, feel cold, loss of appetite)

_____

Bowel Movements (bowel movement scale: 1 = Loose // 6 = Hard)

BM #1 ① ② ③ 4 5 6   BM #3 ① ② ③ 4 5 6
BM #2 ① ② ③ 4 5 6   BM #4 ① ② ③ 4 5 6

BM Notes ▲_____

🩺 **Do you need to call your doctor?** | YES | | NO |

○D **Breakfast** _____

○ **Snack** _____

▢ **Lunch** _____

○ **Snack** _____

🐷 **Dinner** _____

○-○ **Exercise** _____ ⏱ **Time Spent Exercising** _____

✅ **What is one good thing that happened today?**

_____

•1 **What can you do to improve tomorrow?**

_____

▤ **Personal Journal / Notes** (write something about your day or personal thoughts)

_____

_____

_____

_____

_____

_____

_____

Did you know?: Many people with IBD do not even realize when they are running a fever. Low grade fevers do not usually affect daily activities but are good indicators of how well your condition is under control. Check your temperature daily to see how you are doing.

DAY 042

Date _____

Temperature _____ **Weight** _____

Medications Taken Today

1 _____ 2 _____ 3 _____

Pain (Circle most painful moment)

0 1 2 3 4 5 6 7 8 9 10
GOOD   BAD

Types of Pain (circle all that apply)

| DULL | THROBBING | SHARP | CRAMPING |

How long did the pain last? (circle the longest time)

0 1 2 3 4 5 6 7 8 9 10 11 12 13 14 15 16 17 18 19 20 [More +]
Minutes

How many times have you experienced pain today? _____

Sickness Symptoms (cough, sweats, feel cold, loss of appetite)

_____

Bowel Movements (bowel movement scale: 1 = Loose // 6 = Hard)

BM #1 1 2 3 4 5 6   BM #3 1 2 3 4 5 6

BM #2 1 2 3 4 5 6   BM #4 1 2 3 4 5 6

BM Notes _____

Do you need to call your doctor?   YES   NO

Breakfast _____

_____

Snack _____

_____

Lunch _____

_____

Snack _____

_____

Dinner _____

_____

Exercise _____ Time Spent Exercising _____

What is one good thing that happened today?

_____

What can you do to improve tomorrow?

_____

Personal Journal / Notes (write something about your day or personal thoughts)

_____

_____

_____

_____

_____

_____

Date _____

DAY 043

Temperature _____ **Weight** _____

Medications Taken Today

1 _____ 2 _____ 3 _____

Pain (Circle most painful moment)

0   1   2   3   4   5   6   7   8   9   10
GOOD   BAD

Types of Pain (circle all that apply)

DULL | THROBBING | SHARP | CRAMPING

How long did the pain last? (circle the longest time)

0 1 2 3 4 5 6 7 8 9 10 11 12 13 14 15 16 17 18 19 20 More +

Minutes

How many times have you experienced pain today? _____

Sickness Symptoms (cough, sweats, feel cold, loss of appetite)

Bowel Movements (bowel movement scale: 1 = Loose // 6 = Hard)

BM #1 ① ② ③ ④ ⑤ ⑥   BM #3 ① ② ③ ④ ⑤ ⑥
BM #2 ① ② ③ ④ ⑤ ⑥   BM #4 ① ② ③ ④ ⑤ ⑥

BM Notes _____

Do you need to call your doctor?   YES   NO

85

◯▷ **Breakfast** ▸_____

_____

◯ **Snack** ▸_____

_____

▢ **Lunch** ▸_____

_____

◯ **Snack** ▸_____

_____

◯◯ **Dinner** ▸_____

_____

◻◻ **Exercise** ▸_____ ◯ **Time Spent Exercising** ▸_____

✅ **What is one good thing that happened today?**

▸_____

◂🏁 **What can you do to improve tomorrow?**

▸_____

▤ **Personal Journal / Notes** (write something about your day or personal thoughts)

▸_____

_____

_____

_____

_____

_____

_____

_____

Tip: If you are starting to feel under the weather or think maybe your gut just needs a rest, try a bland diet for one day. A bland diet can consist of limited amounts of fish, pureed veggies, pureed low acid fruits, crackers, plain bread, water, and anything else you have found to be very easily digestible.

Date _____

DAY 044

Temperature _____ **Weight** _____

Medications Taken Today

1 _____ 2 _____ 3 _____

Pain (Circle most painful moment)

0 1 2 3 4 5 6 7 8 9 **10**

GOOD   BAD

Types of Pain (circle all that apply)

| DULL | THROBBING | SHARP | CRAMPING |

How long did the pain last? (circle the longest time)

0 1 2 3 4 5 6 7 8 9 10 11 12 13 14 15 16 17 18 19 20 | More +

Minutes

How many times have you experienced pain today? _____

Sickness Symptoms (cough, sweats, feel cold, loss of appetite)

_____

Bowel Movements (bowel movement scale: 1 = Loose // 6 = Hard)

BM #1 **1** **2** **3** 4 5 6   BM #3 **1** **2** 3 4 5 6

BM #2 **1** **2** 3 4 5 6   BM #4 **1** **2** 3 4 5 6

BM Notes _____

Do you need to call your doctor?   YES   NO

◯ **Breakfast** _____

_____

◯ **Snack** _____

_____

▢ **Lunch** _____

_____

◯ **Snack** _____

_____

Dinner _____

_____

Exercise _____ ⏱ **Time Spent Exercising** _____

✔ **What is one good thing that happened today?**

_____

What can you do to improve tomorrow?

_____

Personal Journal / Notes (write something about your day or personal thoughts)

_____

_____

_____

_____

_____

_____

⊕ Famous People with IBD: Frank Fritz, co-star on the History Channel series, American Pickers.

📅 **Date** _____

DAY 045

🌡 **Temperature** _____ ⚖ **Weight** _____

💊 **Medications Taken Today**

1 _____ 2 _____ 3 _____

Pain (Circle most painful moment)

⓪ —— ① —— ② —— ③ —— ④ —— ⑤ —— ⑥ —— ⑦ —— ⑧ —— ⑨ —— ⑩
GOOD   BAD

Types of Pain (circle all that apply)

| DULL | THROBBING | SHARP | CRAMPING |

How long did the pain last? (circle the longest time)

0 1 2 3 4 5 6 7 8 9 10 11 12 13 14 15 16 17 18 19 20 [More +]
Minutes

How many times have you experienced pain today? _____

⚡ **Sickness Symptoms** (cough, sweats, feel cold, loss of appetite)

_____

Bowel Movements (bowel movement scale: 1 = Loose // 6 = Hard)

BM #1 ① ② ③ 4 5 6   BM #3 ① ② 3 4 5 6

BM #2 ① ② 3 4 5 6   BM #4 ① ② 3 4 5 6

BM Notes _____

🩺 **Do you need to call your doctor?** | YES | | NO |

◐ **Breakfast** _____

_____

◉ **Snack** _____

_____

□ **Lunch** _____

_____

◎ **Snack** _____

_____

♞ **Dinner** _____

_____

□-□ **Exercise** _____ ⏲ **Time Spent Exercising** _____

✔ **What is one good thing that happened today?**

_____

✦ **What can you do to improve tomorrow?**

_____

▤ **Personal Journal / Notes** (write something about your day or personal thoughts)

_____

_____

_____

_____

_____

_____

DAY 046

📅 Date _____

🌡 Temperature _____ **⚖ Weight** _____

💊 Medications Taken Today

1 _____ 2 _____ 3 _____

Pain (Circle most painful moment)

0　1　2　3　4　5　6　7　8　9　**10**

GOOD　　　　　　　　　　　　　　　　BAD

Types of Pain (circle all that apply)

| DULL | THROBBING | SHARP | CRAMPING |

How long did the pain last? (circle the longest time)

0　1　2　3　4　5　6　7　8　9　10　11　12　13　14　15　16　17　18　19　20　[More +]

Minutes

How many times have you experienced pain today? _____

⚡ Sickness Symptoms (cough, sweats, feel cold, loss of appetite)

_____

Bowel Movements (bowel movement scale: 1 = Loose // 6 = Hard)

BM #1　1　2　3　4　5　6　　BM #3　1　2　3　4　5　6

BM #2　1　2　3　4　5　6　　BM #4　1　2　3　4　5　6

BM Notes _____

Do you need to call your doctor?　[YES]　[NO]

◯▷ **Breakfast** ▸_____

_____

◉ **Snack** ▸_____

_____

▢ **Lunch** ▸_____

_____

◉ **Snack** ▸_____

_____

🐷 **Dinner** ▸_____

_____

◖▬◗ **Exercise** ▸_____ ⏱ **Time Spent Exercising** ▸_____

✓ **What is one good thing that happened today?**

▸_____

⁕1 **What can you do to improve tomorrow?**

▸_____

▤ **Personal Journal / Notes** (write something about your day or personal thoughts)

▸_____

_____

_____

_____

_____

_____

⊕ Tip: People on corticosteroids should be evaluated by an eye doctor every 6 months for a routine eye examination. This is because corticosteroids increase the risk of eye inflammation, glaucoma, and cataracts.

DAY 047

📅 **Date** _____

🌡 **Temperature** _____   ⚖ **Weight** _____

💊 **Medications Taken Today**

1 _____   2 _____   3 _____

Pain (Circle most painful moment)

0   1   2   3   4   5   6   7   8   9   10
GOOD   BAD

Types of Pain (circle all that apply)

| DULL | THROBBING | SHARP | CRAMPING |

How long did the pain last? (circle the longest time)

0 1 2 3 4 5 6 7 8 9 10 11 12 13 14 15 16 17 18 19 20 [More +]
Minutes

How many times have you experienced pain today? _____

⚡ **Sickness Symptoms** (cough, sweats, feel cold, loss of appetite)

_____

Bowel Movements (bowel movement scale: 1 = Loose // 6 = Hard)

BM #1 ① ② 3 4 5 6   BM #3 ① 2 3 4 5 6

BM #2 ① ② 3 4 5 6   BM #4 ① 2 3 4 5 6

BM Notes _____

🩺 **Do you need to call your doctor?**   YES   NO

◯◗ **Breakfast** ▸_____

_____

◉ **Snack** ▸_____

_____

▢ **Lunch** ▸_____

_____

◉ **Snack** ▸_____

_____

🍗 **Dinner** ▸_____

_____

◻─◻ **Exercise** ▸_____ ⏱ **Time Spent Exercising** ▸_____

✔ **What is one good thing that happened today?**

▸_____

📌 **What can you do to improve tomorrow?**

▸_____

▤ **Personal Journal / Notes** (write something about your day or personal thoughts)

▸_____

_____

_____

_____

_____

_____

_____

> **Tip:** Take your time when choosing what to eat when eating out, and don't be afraid to ask how the food is prepared. Being a little picky at the dinner table may save you some discomfort later on.

📅 **Date** _____

DAY 048

🌡 **Temperature** _____   ⚖ **Weight** _____

💊 **Medications Taken Today**

1 _____   2 _____   3 _____

🩹 **Pain** (Circle most painful moment)

0 — 1 — 2 — 3 — 4 — 5 — 6 — 7 — 8 — 9 — (10)

GOOD   BAD

Types of Pain (circle all that apply)

| DULL | THROBBING | SHARP | CRAMPING |

How long did the pain last? (circle the longest time)

0 1 2 3 4 5 6 7 8 9 10 11 12 13 14 15 16 17 18 19 20 | More + |

Minutes

How many times have you experienced pain today? _____

⚡ **Sickness Symptoms** (cough, sweats, feel cold, loss of appetite)

_____

🫙 **Bowel Movements** (bowel movement scale: 1 = Loose // 6 = Hard)

BM #1 ① ② ③ 4 5 6   BM #3 ① ② ③ 4 5 6

BM #2 ① ② ③ 4 5 6   BM #4 ① ② ③ 4 5 6

BM Notes _____

🩺 **Do you need to call your doctor?** | YES | | NO |

95

◯ **Breakfast** ▶_____

_____

◯ **Snack** ▶_____

_____

◻ **Lunch** ▶_____

_____

◯ **Snack** ▶_____

_____

◯ **Dinner** ▶_____

_____

◻◻ **Exercise** ▶_____ ◯ **Time Spent Exercising** ▶_____

✓ **What is one good thing that happened today?**

▶_____

✦ **What can you do to improve tomorrow?**

▶_____

▦ **Personal Journal / Notes** (write something about your day or personal thoughts)

▶_____

_____

_____

_____

_____

_____

_____

DAY 049

📅 Date _____

🌡️ Temperature _____   ⚖️ Weight _____

💊 **Medications Taken Today**

1 _____   2 _____   3 _____

🩹 **Pain** (Circle most painful moment)

0 1 2 3 4 5 6 7 8 9 **10**

GOOD   BAD

Types of Pain (circle all that apply)

| DULL | THROBBING | SHARP | CRAMPING |

How long did the pain last? (circle the longest time)

0 1 2 3 4 5 6 7 8 9 10 11 12 13 14 15 16 17 18 19 20 [More +]

Minutes

How many times have you experienced pain today? _____

⚡ **Sickness Symptoms** (cough, sweats, feel cold, loss of appetite)

_____

🩸 **Bowel Movements** (bowel movement scale: 1 = Loose // 6 = Hard)

BM #1 1 2 3 4 5 6   BM #3 1 2 3 4 5 6

BM #2 1 2 3 4 5 6   BM #4 1 2 3 4 5 6

BM Notes _____

🩺 **Do you need to call your doctor?**   YES   NO

97

◯⊃ **Breakfast** ▸_____

◯ **Snack** ▸_____
_____

☐ **Lunch** ▸_____
_____

◯ **Snack** ▸_____
_____

🍗 **Dinner** ▸_____
_____

□—□ **Exercise** ▸_____ 🕐 **Time Spent Exercising** ▸_____

✔ **What is one good thing that happened today?**

▸_____

⚐ **What can you do to improve tomorrow?**

▸_____

▤ **Personal Journal / Notes** (write something about your day or personal thoughts)

▸_____
_____
_____
_____
_____
_____
_____

📅 **Date** _____

DAY 050

🌡 **Temperature** _____ 👁 **Weight** _____

💊 **Medications Taken Today**

1 _____ 2 _____ 3 _____

Pain (Circle most painful moment)

⓪ ① ② ③ ④ ⑤ ⑥ ⑦ ⑧ ⑨ ⑩

GOOD   BAD

Types of Pain (circle all that apply)

| DULL | THROBBING | SHARP | CRAMPING |

How long did the pain last? (circle the longest time)

0 1 2 3 4 5 6 7 8 9 10 11 12 13 14 15 16 17 18 19 20 | More + |

Minutes

How many times have you experienced pain today? ▸ _____

⚡ **Sickness Symptoms** (cough, sweats, feel cold, loss of appetite)

_____

Bowel Movements (bowel movement scale: 1 = Loose // 6 = Hard)

BM #1 ① ② ③ 4 5 6   BM #3 ① ② ③ 4 5 6

BM #2 ① ② ③ 4 5 6   BM #4 ① ② ③ 4 5 6

BM Notes ▸ _____

🩺 **Do you need to call your doctor?** | YES | | NO |

◯▷ **Breakfast** _____

_____

◯ **Snack** _____

_____

▢ **Lunch** _____

_____

◯ **Snack** _____

_____

🍗 **Dinner** _____

_____

◻◻ **Exercise** _____   ⏱ **Time Spent Exercising** _____

✅ **What is one good thing that happened today?**

_____

📌 **What can you do to improve tomorrow?**

_____

📋 **Personal Journal / Notes** (write something about your day or personal thoughts)

_____

_____

_____

_____

_____

_____

_____

Do you exercise daily?: If not, plan a walk today during your lunch break for roughly 20 minutes. A little exercise daily can go a long way to increasing energy levels and improving symptoms.

DAY 051

Date _____

Temperature _____ **Weight** _____

Medications Taken Today

1 _____ 2 _____ 3 _____

Pain (Circle most painful moment)

0 1 2 3 4 5 6 7 8 9 10
GOOD   BAD

Types of Pain (circle all that apply)

DULL | THROBBING | SHARP | CRAMPING

How long did the pain last? (circle the longest time)

0 1 2 3 4 5 6 7 8 9 10 11 12 13 14 15 16 17 18 19 20 [More +]
Minutes

How many times have you experienced pain today? _____

Sickness Symptoms (cough, sweats, feel cold, loss of appetite)

Bowel Movements (bowel movement scale: 1 = Loose // 6 = Hard)

BM #1 1 2 3 4 5 6   BM #3 1 2 3 4 5 6
BM #2 1 2 3 4 5 6   BM #4 1 2 3 4 5 6

BM Notes _____

Do you need to call your doctor?   YES   NO

◯ Breakfast _____

◯ Snack _____

◻ Lunch _____

◯ Snack _____

◯ Dinner _____

◻◻ Exercise _____ ◯ Time Spent Exercising _____

✓ **What is one good thing that happened today?**

_____

↵ **What can you do to improve tomorrow?**

_____

▤ **Personal Journal / Notes** (write something about your day or personal thoughts)

_____

_____

_____

_____

_____

_____

31 Date ◣_____

DAY 052

Temperature ◣_____ ◉ **Weight** ◣_____

Medications Taken Today

1 ◣_____ 2 ◣_____ 3 ◣_____

Pain (Circle most painful moment)

0 — 1 — 2 — 3 — 4 — 5 — 6 — 7 — 8 — 9 — ⑩
GOOD   BAD

Types of Pain (circle all that apply)

| DULL | THROBBING | SHARP | CRAMPING |

How long did the pain last? (circle the longest time)

0 1 2 3 4 5 6 7 8 9 10 11 12 13 14 15 16 17 18 19 20 |More +
Minutes

How many times have you experienced pain today? ◣_____

Sickness Symptoms (cough, sweats, feel cold, loss of appetite)

_____

Bowel Movements (bowel movement scale: 1 = Loose // 6 = Hard)

BM #1 ① ② ③ 4 5 6   BM #3 ① ② ③ 4 5 6
BM #2 ① ② ③ 4 5 6   BM #4 ① ② ③ 4 5 6

BM Notes ◣_____

Do you need to call your doctor? | YES | | NO |

103

◯⫘ **Breakfast** ▸_____

◉ **Snack** ▸_____
_____

▢ **Lunch** ▸_____
_____

◉ **Snack** ▸_____
_____

🎧 **Dinner** ▸_____
_____

⊟ **Exercise** ▸_____ 🕐 **Time Spent Exercising** ▸_____

✓ **What is one good thing that happened today?**

▸_____

✦ **What can you do to improve tomorrow?**

▸_____

▤ **Personal Journal / Notes** (write something about your day or personal thoughts)

▸_____
_____
_____
_____
_____
_____
_____

104

DAY 053

📅 **Date** _____

🌡️ **Temperature** _____   ⚖️ **Weight** _____

💊 **Medications Taken Today**

1 _____   2 _____   3 _____

Pain (Circle most painful moment)

0 1 2 3 4 5 6 7 8 9 **10**

GOOD   BAD

Types of Pain (circle all that apply)

| DULL | THROBBING | SHARP | CRAMPING |

How long did the pain last? (circle the longest time)

0 1 2 3 4 5 6 7 8 9 10 11 12 13 14 15 16 17 18 19 20 [More +]

Minutes

How many times have you experienced pain today? _____

⚡ **Sickness Symptoms** (cough, sweats, feel cold, loss of appetite)

_____

🚽 **Bowel Movements** (bowel movement scale: 1 = Loose // 6 = Hard)

BM #1 ① ② ③ ④ ⑤ ⑥   BM #3 ① ② ③ ④ ⑤ ⑥

BM #2 ① ② ③ ④ ⑤ ⑥   BM #4 ① ② ③ ④ ⑤ ⑥

BM Notes _____

🩺 **Do you need to call your doctor?**   YES   NO

◯⊃ **Breakfast**

◯ **Snack**

▢ **Lunch**

◯ **Snack**

🍗 **Dinner**

○-○ **Exercise** _____ 🕐 **Time Spent Exercising**

✅ **What is one good thing that happened today?**

📌 **What can you do to improve tomorrow?**

📄 **Personal Journal / Notes** (write something about your day or personal thoughts)

Famous People with IBD: Chris Conley, singer for Saves the Day.

📅 **Date** ▟_____

DAY 054

🌡 **Temperature** ▟_____ 👁 **Weight** ▟_____

💊 **Medications Taken Today**

1 ▟_____ 2 ▟_____ 3 ▟_____

✚ **Pain** (Circle most painful moment)

0 — 1 — 2 — 3 — 4 — 5 — 6 — 7 — 8 — 9 — 10
GOOD   BAD

Types of Pain (circle all that apply)

| DULL | THROBBING | SHARP | CRAMPING |

How long did the pain last? (circle the longest time)

0 1 2 3 4 5 6 7 8 9 10 11 12 13 14 15 16 17 18 19 20 [More +]
Minutes

How many times have you experienced pain today? ▟_____

⚡ **Sickness Symptoms** (cough, sweats, feel cold, loss of appetite)

_____

🚽 **Bowel Movements** (bowel movement scale: 1 = Loose // 6 = Hard)

BM #1 ① ② ③ 4 5 6   BM #3 ① ② 3 4 5 6

BM #2 ① ② ③ 4 5 6   BM #4 ① ② 3 4 5 6

BM Notes ▟_____

🩺 **Do you need to call your doctor?** | YES | | NO |

107

◯ **Breakfast** _____

_____

◯ **Snack** _____

_____

◻ **Lunch** _____

_____

◯ **Snack** _____

_____

◯ **Dinner** _____

_____

◻–◻ **Exercise** _____ ◯ **Time Spent Exercising** _____

✓ **What is one good thing that happened today?**

_____

⚐ **What can you do to improve tomorrow?**

_____

▤ **Personal Journal / Notes** (write something about your day or personal thoughts)

_____

_____

_____

_____

_____

_____

_____

Did you know?: It is common for adults to experience some lactose intolerance symptoms as they age. This is especially true in people with Crohn's. If you feel you are experiencing more bloating or gas than normal, try reducing your dairy intake to see if symptoms improve. You can also utilize the many lactase additive products available for people with lactose intolerance.

📅 **Date** _____

DAY 055

🌡️ **Temperature** _____   👁️ **Weight** _____

💊 **Medications Taken Today**

1 _____   2 _____   3 _____

Pain (Circle most painful moment)

0 — 1 — 2 — 3 — 4 — 5 — 6 — 7 — 8 — 9 — ⑩
GOOD   BAD

Types of Pain (circle all that apply)

| DULL | THROBBING | SHARP | CRAMPING |

How long did the pain last? (circle the longest time)

0 1 2 3 4 5 6 7 8 9 10 11 12 13 14 15 16 17 18 19 20 [More +]
Minutes

How many times have you experienced pain today? _____

⚡ **Sickness Symptoms** (cough, sweats, feel cold, loss of appetite)

_____

Bowel Movements (bowel movement scale: 1 = Loose // 6 = Hard)

BM #1 ① ② ③ ④ ⑤ ⑥   BM #3 ① ② ③ ④ ⑤ ⑥
BM #2 ① ② ③ ④ ⑤ ⑥   BM #4 ① ② ③ ④ ⑤ ⑥

BM Notes _____

🩺 **Do you need to call your doctor?** | YES | | NO |

🥚 **Breakfast** _____

_____

◉ **Snack** ▸_____

_____

🍞 **Lunch** ▸_____

_____

◉ **Snack** ▸_____

_____

🍗 **Dinner** ▸_____

_____

━ **Exercise** ▸_____ — 🕐 **Time Spent Exercising** ▸_____

✔ **What is one good thing that happened today?**

▸_____

📌 **What can you do to improve tomorrow?**

▸_____

📋 **Personal Journal / Notes** (write something about your day or personal thoughts)

▸_____

_____

_____

_____

_____

_____

_____

📅 **Date** _____

DAY 056

🌡️ **Temperature** _____ ⚖️ **Weight** _____

💊 **Medications Taken Today**

1 _____ 2 _____ 3 _____

Pain (Circle most painful moment)

0 — 1 — 2 — 3 — 4 — 5 — 6 — 7 — 8 — 9 — 10

GOOD   BAD

Types of Pain (circle all that apply)

| DULL | THROBBING | SHARP | CRAMPING |

How long did the pain last? (circle the longest time)

0 1 2 3 4 5 6 7 8 9 10 11 12 13 14 15 16 17 18 19 20 [More +]

Minutes

How many times have you experienced pain today? _____

⚡ **Sickness Symptoms** (cough, sweats, feel cold, loss of appetite)

_____

Bowel Movements (bowel movement scale: 1 = Loose // 6 = Hard)

BM #1 ① ② ③ ④ ⑤ ⑥   BM #3 ① ② ③ ④ ⑤ ⑥

BM #2 ① ② ③ ④ ⑤ ⑥   BM #4 ① ② ③ ④ ⑤ ⑥

BM Notes _____

🩺 **Do you need to call your doctor?**   YES   NO

◯ **Breakfast** _____

◯ **Snack** _____

◻ **Lunch** _____

◯ **Snack** _____

◯ **Dinner** _____

◻◻ **Exercise** _____ ◷ **Time Spent Exercising** _____

✅ **What is one good thing that happened today?**

_____

📌 **What can you do to improve tomorrow?**

_____

📄 **Personal Journal / Notes** (write something about your day or personal thoughts)

_____

_____

_____

_____

_____

_____

📅 **Date** ▸_____

DAY 057

🌡️ **Temperature** ▸_____   👁️ **Weight** ▸_____

💊 **Medications Taken Today**

1 ▸_____   2 ▸_____   3 ▸_____

Pain (Circle most painful moment)

0 — 1 — 2 — 3 — 4 — 5 — 6 — 7 — 8 — 9 — 10
GOOD   BAD

Types of Pain (circle all that apply)

| DULL | THROBBING | SHARP | CRAMPING |

How long did the pain last? (circle the longest time)

0 1 2 3 4 5 6 7 8 9 10 11 12 13 14 15 16 17 18 19 20 [More +]
Minutes

How many times have you experienced pain today? ▸_____

⚡ **Sickness Symptoms** (cough, sweats, feel cold, loss of appetite)

⚗️ **Bowel Movements** (bowel movement scale: 1 = Loose // 6 = Hard)

BM #1 ① ② ③ ④ ⑤ ⑥   BM #3 ① ② ③ ④ ⑤ ⑥

BM #2 ① ② ③ ④ ⑤ ⑥   BM #4 ① ② ③ ④ ⑤ ⑥

BM Notes ▸_____

🩺 **Do you need to call your doctor?**   YES   NO

113

◯⊃ **Breakfast** ▸ _____

_____

◉ **Snack** ▸ _____

_____

▢ **Lunch** ▸ _____

_____

◉ **Snack** ▸ _____

_____

🐑 **Dinner** ▸ _____

_____

◻–◻ **Exercise** ▸ _____ 🕐 **Time Spent Exercising** ▸ _____

✅ **What is one good thing that happened today?**

▸ _____

+1 **What can you do to improve tomorrow?**

▸ _____

📋 **Personal Journal / Notes** (write something about your day or personal thoughts)

▸ _____

_____

_____

_____

_____

_____

_____

Did you know?: Protein depletion is a common side effect of IBD. Some symptoms of protein depletion can be swelling, stunted growth, bone pain, and an absence of menstrual periods.

📅 **Date** _____

DAY 058

🌡 **Temperature** _____   👁 **Weight** _____

💊 **Medications Taken Today**

1 _____   2 _____   3 _____

Pain (Circle most painful moment)

(0)—(1)—(2)—(3)—(4)—(5)—(6)—(7)—(8)—(9)—(10)
GOOD   BAD

Types of Pain (circle all that apply)

| DULL | THROBBING | SHARP | CRAMPING |

How long did the pain last? (circle the longest time)

0 1 2 3 4 5 6 7 8 9 10 11 12 13 14 15 16 17 18 19 20 [More +]
Minutes

How many times have you experienced pain today? _____

⚡ **Sickness Symptoms** (cough, sweats, feel cold, loss of appetite)

_____

Bowel Movements (bowel movement scale: 1 = Loose // 6 = Hard)

BM #1 ① ② ③ ④ ⑤ ⑥   BM #3 ① ② ③ ④ ⑤ ⑥

BM #2 ① ② ③ ④ ⑤ ⑥   BM #4 ① ② ③ ④ ⑤ ⑥

BM Notes _____

🩺 **Do you need to call your doctor?** | YES | | NO |

◯▷ **Breakfast** ▸_____

◉ **Snack** ▸_____

▢ **Lunch** ▸_____

◉ **Snack** ▸_____

🐑 **Dinner** ▸_____

〇–〇 **Exercise** ▸_____ ⏱ **Time Spent Exercising** ▸_____

✔ **What is one good thing that happened today?**

▸_____

◀ **What can you do to improve tomorrow?**

▸_____

▤ **Personal Journal / Notes** (write something about your day or personal thoughts)

▸_____

_____

_____

_____

_____

_____

_____

_____

Tip: If you have a hard time with needles, try icing the area to reduce the pain or ask your doctor about a skin numbing agent such as lidocaine.

Date _____

DAY 059

Temperature _____ **Weight** _____

Medications Taken Today

1 _____ 2 _____ 3 _____

Pain (Circle most painful moment)

0 1 2 3 4 5 6 7 8 9 **10**

GOOD   BAD

Types of Pain (circle all that apply)

| DULL | THROBBING | SHARP | CRAMPING |

How long did the pain last? (circle the longest time)

0 1 2 3 4 5 6 7 8 9 10 11 12 13 14 15 16 17 18 19 20 [More +]

Minutes

How many times have you experienced pain today? _____

Sickness Symptoms (cough, sweats, feel cold, loss of appetite)

Bowel Movements (bowel movement scale: 1 = Loose // 6 = Hard)

BM #1 **1** **2** 3 4 5 6   BM #3 **1** **2** 3 4 5 6

BM #2 **1** **2** **3** 4 5 6   BM #4 **1** **2** **3** 4 5 6

BM Notes _____

Do you need to call your doctor?   YES   NO

◯ **Breakfast** ▶_____

_____

◉ **Snack** ▶_____

_____

☐ **Lunch** ▶_____

_____

◉ **Snack** ▶_____

_____

🎧 **Dinner** ▶_____

_____

▢–▢ **Exercise** ▶_____   🕐 **Time Spent Exercising** ▶_____

✓ **What is one good thing that happened today?**

▶_____

+1 **What can you do to improve tomorrow?**

▶_____

▤ **Personal Journal / Notes** (write something about your day or personal thoughts)

▶_____

_____

_____

_____

_____

_____

_____

⊕ Famous People with IBD: Jim Myers, AKA: George "The Animal" Steele, Professional WWE Wrestler and WWE Hall Of Fame inductee.

📅 Date _____

DAY 060

🌡 Temperature _____   **⚖ Weight** _____

Medications Taken Today

1 _____   2 _____   3 _____

Pain (Circle most painful moment)

⓪ ① ② ③ ④ ⑤ ⑥ ⑦ ⑧ ⑨ ⑩
GOOD   BAD

Types of Pain (circle all that apply)

| DULL | THROBBING | SHARP | CRAMPING |

How long did the pain last? (circle the longest time)

0 1 2 3 4 5 6 7 8 9 10 11 12 13 14 15 16 17 18 19 20 More +
Minutes

How many times have you experienced pain today? _____

⚡ Sickness Symptoms (cough, sweats, feel cold, loss of appetite)

Bowel Movements (bowel movement scale: 1 = Loose // 6 = Hard)

BM #1 ① ② ③ ④ ⑤ ⑥   BM #3 ① ② ③ ④ ⑤ ⑥
BM #2 ① ② ③ ④ ⑤ ⑥   BM #4 ① ② ③ ④ ⑤ ⑥

BM Notes _____

Do you need to call your doctor?   YES   NO

◯ **Breakfast** _____

_____

◉ **Snack** _____

_____

▢ **Lunch** _____

_____

◉ **Snack** _____

_____

Dinner _____

_____

Exercise _____   ◷ **Time Spent Exercising** _____

✓ **What is one good thing that happened today?**

_____

What can you do to improve tomorrow?

_____

▤ **Personal Journal / Notes** (write something about your day or personal thoughts)

_____

_____

_____

_____

_____

_____

_____

Tip: If you are experiencing a sudden loss in appetite for more than 1 or 2 days, call your doctor immediately. Many times, loss of appetite is a symptom of a flare or a blockage. Addressing it early can reduce the risks of needing to take extreme measures.

DAY 061

📅 **Date** _____

🌡️ **Temperature** _____   ⚖️ **Weight** _____

💊 **Medications Taken Today**

1 _____ 2 _____ 3 _____

🩹 **Pain** (Circle most painful moment)

(0)—(1)—(2)—(3)—(4)—(5)—(6)—(7)—(8)—(9)—(10)
GOOD   BAD

Types of Pain (circle all that apply)

| DULL | | THROBBING | | SHARP | | CRAMPING |

How long did the pain last? (circle the longest time)

0 1 2 3 4 5 6 7 8 9 10 11 12 13 14 15 16 17 18 19 20 [More +]
Minutes

How many times have you experienced pain today? _____

⚡ **Sickness Symptoms** (cough, sweats, feel cold, loss of appetite)

_____

Bowel Movements (bowel movement scale: 1 = Loose // 6 = Hard)

BM #1 ① ② ③ ④ ⑤ ⑥   BM #3 ① ② ③ ④ ⑤ ⑥
BM #2 ① ② ③ ④ ⑤ ⑥   BM #4 ① ② ③ ④ ⑤ ⑥

BM Notes _____

🩺 **Do you need to call your doctor?**   YES   NO

○ **Breakfast**

○ **Snack**

○ **Lunch**

○ **Snack**

○ **Dinner**

○ **Exercise** ⌚ **Time Spent Exercising**

✔ **What is one good thing that happened today?**

+1 **What can you do to improve tomorrow?**

▤ **Personal Journal / Notes** (write something about your day or personal thoughts)

Tip: If you are experiencing cramps or abdominal pain, try applying a warm compress to your abdomen and finding the most comfortable position possible. This may help to alleviate some discomfort.

Date _____

DAY 062

Temperature _____   **Weight** _____

Medications Taken Today

1 _____   2 _____   3 _____

Pain (Circle most painful moment)

(0) (1) (2) (3) (4) (5) (6) (7) (8) (9) (10)
GOOD   BAD

Types of Pain (circle all that apply)

| DULL | THROBBING | SHARP | CRAMPING |

How long did the pain last? (circle the longest time)

0 1 2 3 4 5 6 7 8 9 10 11 12 13 14 15 16 17 18 19 20 [More +]
Minutes

How many times have you experienced pain today? _____

Sickness Symptoms (cough, sweats, feel cold, loss of appetite)

Bowel Movements (bowel movement scale: 1 = Loose // 6 = Hard)

BM #1 ① ② ③ ④ ⑤ ⑥   BM #3 ① ② ③ ④ ⑤ ⑥

BM #2 ① ② ③ ④ ⑤ ⑥   BM #4 ① ② ③ ④ ⑤ ⑥

BM Notes _____

Do you need to call your doctor?   YES   NO

◐ **Breakfast** _____
_____

◉ **Snack** _____
_____

▢ **Lunch** _____
_____

◉ **Snack** _____
_____

🍗 **Dinner** _____
_____

▭ **Exercise** _____   ◷ **Time Spent Exercising** _____

✅ **What is one good thing that happened today?**
_____

➕1 **What can you do to improve tomorrow?**
_____

▤ **Personal Journal / Notes** (write something about your day or personal thoughts)
_____
_____
_____
_____
_____
_____
_____

⊕ Famous People with IBD: Beth Orton, a famous British singer/songwriter.

📅 **Date** ↳ _____

DAY 063

🌡 **Temperature** ↳ _____   ⚖ **Weight** ↳ _____

💊 **Medications Taken Today**

1 ↳ _____   2 ↳ _____   3 ↳ _____

🩹 **Pain** (Circle most painful moment)

(0) (1) (2) (3) (4) (5) (6) (7) (8) (9) (10)
GOOD   BAD

Types of Pain (circle all that apply)

| DULL | THROBBING | SHARP | CRAMPING |

How long did the pain last? (circle the longest time)

0 1 2 3 4 5 6 7 8 9 10 11 12 13 14 15 16 17 18 19 20 [More +]
Minutes

How many times have you experienced pain today? ↳ _____

⚡ **Sickness Symptoms** (cough, sweats, feel cold, loss of appetite)

_____

🚽 **Bowel Movements** (bowel movement scale: 1 = Loose // 6 = Hard)

BM #1 ① ② ③ ④ ⑤ ⑥   BM #3 ① ② ③ ④ ⑤ ⑥

BM #2 ① ② ③ ④ ⑤ ⑥   BM #4 ① ② ③ ④ ⑤ ⑥

BM Notes ↳ _____

🩺 **Do you need to call your doctor?** | YES | | NO |

○ **Breakfast** _____

◉ **Snack** _____

☐ **Lunch** _____

◉ **Snack** _____

🐑 **Dinner** _____

○─○ **Exercise** _____ ⏱ **Time Spent Exercising** _____

✓ **What is one good thing that happened today?**

_____

+1 **What can you do to improve tomorrow?**

_____

📋 **Personal Journal / Notes** (write something about your day or personal thoughts)

_____

_____

_____

_____

_____

_____

_____

Date

DAY 064

Temperature _____ **Weight** _____

Medications Taken Today

1 _____ 2 _____ 3 _____

Pain (Circle most painful moment)

⓪ ① ② ③ ④ ⑤ ⑥ ⑦ ⑧ ⑨ ⑩

GOOD   BAD

Types of Pain (circle all that apply)

| DULL | THROBBING | SHARP | CRAMPING |

How long did the pain last? (circle the longest time)

0 1 2 3 4 5 6 7 8 9 10 11 12 13 14 15 16 17 18 19 20 More +

Minutes

How many times have you experienced pain today? _____

Sickness Symptoms (cough, sweats, feel cold, loss of appetite)

Bowel Movements (bowel movement scale: 1 = Loose // 6 = Hard)

BM #1 ① ② ③ ④ ⑤ ⑥   BM #3 ① ② ③ ④ ⑤ ⑥

BM #2 ① ② ③ ④ ⑤ ⑥   BM #4 ① ② ③ ④ ⑤ ⑥

BM Notes _____

Do you need to call your doctor?   YES   NO

○○ Breakfast _____

⊙ Snack _____

□ Lunch _____

⊙ Snack _____

🐑 Dinner _____

○-○ Exercise _____ ⏱ Time Spent Exercising _____

✅ **What is one good thing that happened today?**

_____

📌 **What can you do to improve tomorrow?**

_____

📋 **Personal Journal / Notes** (write something about your day or personal thoughts)

_____

_____

_____

_____

_____

_____

⊕ Tip: Eat 5 smaller meals a day. If that isn't feasible, try eating 3 medium-sized meals and 2 small meals or snacks a day.

📅 **Date** ↳ _____

DAY 065

🌡 **Temperature** ↳ _____   👁 **Weight** ↳ _____

💊 **Medications Taken Today**

1 ↳ _____   2 ↳ _____   3 ↳ _____

🩹 **Pain** (Circle most painful moment)

(0) — (1) — (2) — (3) — (4) — (5) — (6) — (7) — (8) — (9) — (10)

GOOD   BAD

Types of Pain (circle all that apply)

| DULL | THROBBING | SHARP | CRAMPING |

How long did the pain last? (circle the longest time)

0 1 2 3 4 5 6 7 8 9 10 11 12 13 14 15 16 17 18 19 20 [More +]

Minutes

How many times have you experienced pain today? ↳ _____

⚡ **Sickness Symptoms** (cough, sweats, feel cold, loss of appetite)

_____

🧫 **Bowel Movements** (bowel movement scale: 1 = Loose // 6 = Hard)

BM #1 **①** **②** **③** **④** **⑤** **⑥**   BM #3 **①** **②** **③** **④** **⑤** **⑥**

BM #2 **①** **②** **③** **④** **⑤** **⑥**   BM #4 **①** **②** **③** **④** **⑤** **⑥**

BM Notes ↳ _____

🩺 **Do you need to call your doctor?** | YES | | NO |

◐ **Breakfast** ►_____

_____

◉ **Snack** ►_____

_____

⬜ **Lunch** ►_____

_____

◉ **Snack** ►_____

_____

🍗 **Dinner** ►_____

_____

☐─☐ **Exercise** ►_____ 🕐 **Time Spent Exercising** ►_____

✓ **What is one good thing that happened today?**

►_____

+1 **What can you do to improve tomorrow?**

►_____

▤ **Personal Journal / Notes** (write something about your day or personal thoughts)

►_____

_____

_____

_____

_____

_____

_____

📅 **Date** _____

DAY 066

🌡 **Temperature** _____   🔘 **Weight** _____

💊 **Medications Taken Today**

1 _____   2 _____   3 _____

🩹 **Pain** (Circle most painful moment)

(0) (1) (2) (3) (4) (5) (6) (7) (8) (9) (10)

GOOD   BAD

Types of Pain (circle all that apply)

| DULL | THROBBING | SHARP | CRAMPING |

How long did the pain last? (circle the longest time)

0 1 2 3 4 5 6 7 8 9 10 11 12 13 14 15 16 17 18 19 20 [More +]

Minutes

How many times have you experienced pain today? _____

⚡ **Sickness Symptoms** (cough, sweats, feel cold, loss of appetite)

_____

🍶 **Bowel Movements** (bowel movement scale: 1 = Loose // 6 = Hard)

BM #1 ❶ ❷ ❸ ❹ ❺ ❻   BM #3 ❶ ❷ ❸ ❹ ❺ ❻

BM #2 ❶ ❷ ❸ ❹ ❺ ❻   BM #4 ❶ ❷ ❸ ❹ ❺ ❻

BM Notes _____

🩺 **Do you need to call your doctor?**   [YES]   [NO]

Breakfast ▶_____

_____

Snack ▶_____

_____

Lunch ▶_____

_____

Snack ▶_____

_____

Dinner ▶_____

_____

Exercise ▶_____ Time Spent Exercising ▶_____

✔ **What is one good thing that happened today?**

▶_____

+1 **What can you do to improve tomorrow?**

▶_____

Personal Journal / Notes (write something about your day or personal thoughts)

▶_____

_____

_____

_____

_____

_____

_____

Tip: Stay Social! Multiple studies have proven that staying social can help you to feel better, recover more quickly, and keep a positive outlook. Even if you don't feel like eating, just drinking tea or water can still keep you as a part of the social activity.

Date

DAY 067

Temperature _____   **Weight** _____

Medications Taken Today

1 _____   2 _____   3 _____

Pain (Circle most painful moment)

0 1 2 3 4 5 6 7 8 9 10
GOOD   BAD

Types of Pain (circle all that apply)

DULL | THROBBING | SHARP | CRAMPING

How long did the pain last? (circle the longest time)

0 1 2 3 4 5 6 7 8 9 10 11 12 13 14 15 16 17 18 19 20 [More +]
Minutes

How many times have you experienced pain today? _____

Sickness Symptoms (cough, sweats, feel cold, loss of appetite)

Bowel Movements (bowel movement scale: 1 = Loose // 6 = Hard)

BM #1 1 2 3 4 5 6   BM #3 1 2 3 4 5 6

BM #2 1 2 3 4 5 6   BM #4 1 2 3 4 5 6

BM Notes _____

Do you need to call your doctor?   YES   NO

◯▷ **Breakfast** _____

◉ **Snack** _____

▢ **Lunch** _____

◉ **Snack** _____

🍗 **Dinner** _____

▢—▢ **Exercise** _____ 🕐 **Time Spent Exercising** _____

✅ **What is one good thing that happened today?**
_____

+1 **What can you do to improve tomorrow?**
_____

📋 **Personal Journal / Notes** (write something about your day or personal thoughts)
_____
_____
_____
_____
_____
_____
_____

Tip: Whenever you are about to have a procedure done or receive a new medication, it is important to understand the reasons for it. Ask your doctor simple why, what and how questions such as "Why is this being done?"; "What should the expected benefit be?"; and "How will this help me?"

DAY 068

📅 **Date** _____

🌡️ **Temperature** _____   👁️ **Weight** _____

💊 **Medications Taken Today**

1 _____   2 _____   3 _____

Pain (Circle most painful moment)

0　1　2　3　4　5　6　7　8　9　**10**
GOOD　　　　　　　　　　　　　　　　BAD

Types of Pain (circle all that apply)

DULL | THROBBING | SHARP | CRAMPING

How long did the pain last? (circle the longest time)

0　1　2　3　4　5　6　7　8　9　10　11　12　13　14　15　16　17　18　19　20　[More +]
Minutes

How many times have you experienced pain today? _____

⚡ **Sickness Symptoms** (cough, sweats, feel cold, loss of appetite)

_____

Bowel Movements (bowel movement scale: 1 = Loose // 6 = Hard)

BM #1　①　②　③　④　⑤　⑥　　　BM #3　①　②　③　④　⑤　⑥
BM #2　①　②　③　④　⑤　⑥　　　BM #4　①　②　③　④　⑤　⑥

BM Notes _____

🩺 **Do you need to call your doctor?**　[YES]　[NO]

Breakfast _____
_____

Snack _____
_____

Lunch _____
_____

Snack _____
_____

Dinner _____
_____

Exercise _____ Time Spent Exercising _____

What is one good thing that happened today?

_____

What can you do to improve tomorrow?

_____

Personal Journal / Notes (write something about your day or personal thoughts)

_____
_____
_____
_____
_____
_____
_____
_____

Did you know?: Some people with Crohn's may experience eye inflammation. This is less common but occurs most commonly during a flare. This should be reported to your doctor immediately upon occurrence.

📅 Date _____

DAY 069

🌡 Temperature _____   **⚖ Weight** _____

💊 Medications Taken Today

1 _____   2 _____   3 _____

Pain (Circle most painful moment)

0 — 1 — 2 — 3 — 4 — 5 — 6 — 7 — 8 — 9 — **(10)**

GOOD   BAD

Types of Pain (circle all that apply)

| DULL | THROBBING | SHARP | CRAMPING |

How long did the pain last? (circle the longest time)

0 1 2 3 4 5 6 7 8 9 10 11 12 13 14 15 16 17 18 19 20 [More +]

Minutes

How many times have you experienced pain today? _____

Sickness Symptoms (cough, sweats, feel cold, loss of appetite)

_____

Bowel Movements (bowel movement scale: 1 = Loose // 6 = Hard)

BM #1 **①** **②** 3 4 5 6   BM #3 **①** **②** 3 4 5 6

BM #2 **①** **②** 3 4 5 6   BM #4 **①** **②** 3 4 5 6

BM Notes _____

Do you need to call your doctor?   YES   NO

Breakfast _____

Snack _____

Lunch _____

Snack _____

Dinner _____

Exercise _____ Time Spent Exercising _____

What is one good thing that happened today?

_____

What can you do to improve tomorrow?

_____

Personal Journal / Notes (write something about your day or personal thoughts)

_____

_____

_____

_____

_____

_____

⊕ Famous People with IBD: Rocker McCready, lead guitarist for Pearl Jam.

📅 **Date** _____ **DAY 070**

🌡 **Temperature** _____   ⚖ **Weight** _____

💊 **Medications Taken Today**

1_____   2_____   3_____

Pain (Circle most painful moment)

0 1 2 3 4 5 6 7 8 9 10
GOOD   BAD

Types of Pain (circle all that apply)

DULL | **THROBBING** | **SHARP** | **CRAMPING**

How long did the pain last? (circle the longest time)

0 1 2 3 4 5 6 7 8 9 10 11 12 13 14 15 16 17 18 19 20 [More +]
Minutes

How many times have you experienced pain today? _____

⚡ **Sickness Symptoms** (cough, sweats, feel cold, loss of appetite)

Bowel Movements (bowel movement scale: 1 = Loose // 6 = Hard)

BM #1 ① ② ③ ④ ⑤ ⑥   BM #3 ① ② ③ ④ ⑤ ⑥
BM #2 ① ② ③ ④ ⑤ ⑥   BM #4 ① ② ③ ④ ⑤ ⑥

BM Notes _____

🩺 **Do you need to call your doctor?**   YES   NO

ⓑ Breakfast ▸_____

_____

◔ Snack ▸_____

_____

▢ Lunch ▸_____

_____

◔ Snack ▸_____

_____

🍗 Dinner ▸_____

_____

⊐⊏ Exercise ▸_____   🕐 Time Spent Exercising ▸_____

✔ **What is one good thing that happened today?**

▸_____

➕ **What can you do to improve tomorrow?**

▸_____

▤ **Personal Journal / Notes** (write something about your day or personal thoughts)

▸_____

_____

_____

_____

_____

_____

_____

Date _____

DAY 071

Temperature _____   **Weight** _____

Medications Taken Today

1 _____   2 _____   3 _____

Pain (Circle most painful moment)

⓪ ① ② ③ ④ ⑤ ⑥ ⑦ ⑧ ⑨ ⑩
GOOD   BAD

Types of Pain (circle all that apply)

| DULL | THROBBING | SHARP | CRAMPING |

How long did the pain last? (circle the longest time)

0 1 2 3 4 5 6 7 8 9 10 11 12 13 14 15 16 17 18 19 20 More +
Minutes

How many times have you experienced pain today? _____

Sickness Symptoms (cough, sweats, feel cold, loss of appetite)

Bowel Movements (bowel movement scale: 1 = Loose // 6 = Hard)

BM #1 ① ② ③ ④ ⑤ ⑥   BM #3 ① ② ③ ④ ⑤ ⑥

BM #2 ① ② ③ ④ ⑤ ⑥   BM #4 ① ② ③ ④ ⑤ ⑥

BM Notes _____

Do you need to call your doctor?   YES   NO

◑ Breakfast ▬▬▬▬▬▬▬▬▬▬▬▬▬▬▬▬▬▬▬▬▬▬▬▬▬▬▬▬

▬▬▬▬▬▬▬▬▬▬▬▬▬▬▬▬▬▬▬▬▬▬▬▬▬▬▬

◉ Snack ▬▬▬▬▬▬▬▬▬▬▬▬▬▬▬▬▬▬▬▬▬▬▬▬▬

▬▬▬▬▬▬▬▬▬▬▬▬▬▬▬▬▬▬▬▬▬▬▬▬▬▬▬

▢ Lunch ▬▬▬▬▬▬▬▬▬▬▬▬▬▬▬▬▬▬▬▬▬▬▬▬▬

▬▬▬▬▬▬▬▬▬▬▬▬▬▬▬▬▬▬▬▬▬▬▬▬▬▬▬

◉ Snack ▬▬▬▬▬▬▬▬▬▬▬▬▬▬▬▬▬▬▬▬▬▬▬▬▬

▬▬▬▬▬▬▬▬▬▬▬▬▬▬▬▬▬▬▬▬▬▬▬▬▬▬▬

🐑 Dinner ▬▬▬▬▬▬▬▬▬▬▬▬▬▬▬▬▬▬▬▬▬▬▬▬

▬▬▬▬▬▬▬▬▬▬▬▬▬▬▬▬▬▬▬▬▬▬▬▬▬▬▬

⊡─O Exercise ▬▬▬▬▬▬▬▬▬   ⏱ Time Spent Exercising ▬▬▬▬▬

✅ **What is one good thing that happened today?**

▬▬▬▬▬▬▬▬▬▬▬▬▬▬▬▬▬▬▬▬▬▬▬▬▬▬▬▬

+1 **What can you do to improve tomorrow?**

▬▬▬▬▬▬▬▬▬▬▬▬▬▬▬▬▬▬▬▬▬▬▬▬▬▬▬▬

▤ **Personal Journal / Notes** (write something about your day or personal thoughts)

▬▬▬▬▬▬▬▬▬▬▬▬▬▬▬▬▬▬▬▬▬▬▬▬▬▬▬▬

▬▬▬▬▬▬▬▬▬▬▬▬▬▬▬▬▬▬▬▬▬▬▬▬▬▬▬▬

▬▬▬▬▬▬▬▬▬▬▬▬▬▬▬▬▬▬▬▬▬▬▬▬▬▬▬▬

▬▬▬▬▬▬▬▬▬▬▬▬▬▬▬▬▬▬▬▬▬▬▬▬▬▬▬▬

▬▬▬▬▬▬▬▬▬▬▬▬▬▬▬▬▬▬▬▬▬▬▬▬▬▬▬▬

▬▬▬▬▬▬▬▬▬▬▬▬▬▬▬▬▬▬▬▬▬▬▬▬▬▬▬▬

> **Did you know?:** Canker sores inside the mouth are common in people with Crohn's and are usually more present during a flare. Ask your doctor about topical ointments that can be used for treatment.

Date _____

DAY 072

Temperature _____   **Weight** _____

Medications Taken Today

1 _____   2 _____   3 _____

Pain (Circle most painful moment)

0 — 1 — 2 — 3 — 4 — 5 — 6 — 7 — 8 — 9 — **10**

GOOD   BAD

Types of Pain (circle all that apply)

DULL | **THROBBING** | **SHARP** | **CRAMPING**

How long did the pain last? (circle the longest time)

0 1 2 3 4 5 6 7 8 9 10 11 12 13 14 15 16 17 18 19 20 More +

Minutes

How many times have you experienced pain today? _____

Sickness Symptoms (cough, sweats, feel cold, loss of appetite)

_____

Bowel Movements (bowel movement scale: 1 = Loose // 6 = Hard)

BM #1 **1** **2** 3 4 5 6   BM #3 **1** 2 3 4 5 6

BM #2 **1** **2** 3 4 5 6   BM #4 **1** **2** 3 4 5 6

BM Notes _____

Do you need to call your doctor?   YES   NO

◯▷ **Breakfast** _____

◯ **Snack** _____

▢ **Lunch** _____

◯ **Snack** _____

🍗 **Dinner** _____

◘-◘ **Exercise** _____ 🕐 **Time Spent Exercising** _____

✅ **What is one good thing that happened today?**

_____

📌 **What can you do to improve tomorrow?**

_____

📋 **Personal Journal / Notes** (write something about your day or personal thoughts)

_____

_____

_____

_____

_____

_____

_____

Tip: Make it a game to find new and unusual foods that can help you to reach your nutritional goals. This can help expand your available menus and help to spice up the dinner table. Remember, introducing new foods should be done in a controlled manner and recorded to see if there are any negative effects.

DAY 073

📅 **Date** _____

🌡️ **Temperature** _____   ⚖️ **Weight** _____

💊 **Medications Taken Today**

1 _____   2 _____   3 _____

🩹 **Pain** (Circle most painful moment)

⓪ ① ② ③ ④ ⑤ ⑥ ⑦ ⑧ ⑨ ⑩

GOOD   BAD

Types of Pain (circle all that apply)

| DULL | THROBBING | SHARP | CRAMPING |

How long did the pain last? (circle the longest time)

0 1 2 3 4 5 6 7 8 9 10 11 12 13 14 15 16 17 18 19 20 [More +]

Minutes

How many times have you experienced pain today? _____

⚡ **Sickness Symptoms** (cough, sweats, feel cold, loss of appetite)

_____

🚽 **Bowel Movements** (bowel movement scale: 1 = Loose // 6 = Hard)

BM #1 ① ② ③ ④ ⑤ ⑥   BM #3 ① ② ③ ④ ⑤ ⑥

BM #2 ① ② ③ ④ ⑤ ⑥   BM #4 ① ② ③ ④ ⑤ ⑥

BM Notes _____

🩺 **Do you need to call your doctor?**   YES   NO

○ **Breakfast** ▶ _____

⊙ **Snack** ▶ _____

▢ **Lunch** ▶ _____

⊙ **Snack** ▶ _____

🐔 **Dinner** ▶ _____

⊏⊐ **Exercise** ▶ _____ ⏱ **Time Spent Exercising** ▶ _____

✔ **What is one good thing that happened today?**

▶ _____

✦ **What can you do to improve tomorrow?**

▶ _____

▤ **Personal Journal / Notes** (write something about your day or personal thoughts)

▶ _____

_____

_____

_____

_____

_____

DAY 074

📅 Date _____

🌡 Temperature _____   👁 Weight _____

💊 **Medications Taken Today**

1 _____   2 _____   3 _____

Pain (Circle most painful moment)

0 — 1 — 2 — 3 — 4 — 5 — 6 — 7 — 8 — 9 — **10**

GOOD   BAD

Types of Pain (circle all that apply)

| DULL | THROBBING | SHARP | CRAMPING |

How long did the pain last? (circle the longest time)

0 1 2 3 4 5 6 7 8 9 10 11 12 13 14 15 16 17 18 19 20 [More +]

Minutes

How many times have you experienced pain today? _____

⚡ **Sickness Symptoms** (cough, sweats, feel cold, loss of appetite)

_____

Bowel Movements (bowel movement scale: 1 = Loose // 6 = Hard)

BM #1 ① ② ③ ④ ⑤ ⑥   BM #3 ① ② ③ ④ ⑤ ⑥

BM #2 ① ② ③ ④ ⑤ ⑥   BM #4 ① ② ③ ④ ⑤ ⑥

BM Notes _____

🩺 **Do you need to call your doctor?**   YES   NO

◯▷ **Breakfast** ▸_____

_____

◉ **Snack** ▸_____

_____

▢ **Lunch** ▸_____

_____

◉ **Snack** ▸_____

_____

🐔 **Dinner** ▸_____

_____

▥ **Exercise** ▸_____ ⏱ **Time Spent Exercising** ▸_____

✓ **What is one good thing that happened today?**

▸_____

+1 **What can you do to improve tomorrow?**

▸_____

▤ **Personal Journal / Notes** (write something about your day or personal thoughts)

▸_____

_____

_____

_____

_____

_____

_____

Tip: When going out in public, carry a pack of tissues just in case the place you are visiting is not well stocked with toilet paper.

📅 **Date** _____

DAY 075

🌡 **Temperature** _____ 👁 **Weight** _____

💊 **Medications Taken Today**

1 _____ 2 _____ 3 _____

Pain (Circle most painful moment)

0 — 1 — 2 — 3 — 4 — 5 — 6 — 7 — 8 — 9 — **10**

GOOD   BAD

Types of Pain (circle all that apply)

| DULL | THROBBING | SHARP | CRAMPING |

How long did the pain last? (circle the longest time)

0 1 2 3 4 5 6 7 8 9 10 11 12 13 14 15 16 17 18 19 20 More +

Minutes

How many times have you experienced pain today? _____

⚡ **Sickness Symptoms** (cough, sweats, feel cold, loss of appetite)

_____

Bowel Movements (bowel movement scale: 1 = Loose // 6 = Hard)

BM #1 **1** **2** 3 4 5 6   BM #3 **1** 2 3 4 5 6

BM #2 **1** **2** 3 4 5 6   BM #4 **1** 2 3 4 5 6

BM Notes _____

🩺 **Do you need to call your doctor?**   [YES]   [NO]

◯▷ **Breakfast** ▸_____

_____

◉ **Snack** ▸_____

_____

▢ **Lunch** ▸_____

_____

◉ **Snack** ▸_____

_____

🍗 **Dinner** ▸_____

_____

◻─◻ **Exercise** ▸_____ 🕐 **Time Spent Exercising** ▸_____

✔ **What is one good thing that happened today?**

▸_____

📄 **What can you do to improve tomorrow?**

▸_____

▤ **Personal Journal / Notes** (write something about your day or personal thoughts)

▸_____

_____

_____

_____

_____

_____

_____

Did you know?: Adding supplements to your vitamin intake may help to stabilize your weight and give you added energy. This is because your body may not be able to absorb specific nutrients as easily as others. Since each case is different, discuss which supplements may be beneficial to you with your doctor.

DAY 076

Date

Temperature   **Weight**

Medications Taken Today

1   2   3

Pain (Circle most painful moment)

0 1 2 3 4 5 6 7 8 9 10
GOOD   BAD

Types of Pain (circle all that apply)

DULL | THROBBING | SHARP | CRAMPING

How long did the pain last? (circle the longest time)

0 1 2 3 4 5 6 7 8 9 10 11 12 13 14 15 16 17 18 19 20 More +
Minutes

How many times have you experienced pain today?

Sickness Symptoms (cough, sweats, feel cold, loss of appetite)

Bowel Movements (bowel movement scale: 1 = Loose // 6 = Hard)

BM #1 ① ② ③ ④ ⑤ ⑥   BM #3 ① ② ③ ④ ⑤ ⑥

BM #2 ① ② ③ ④ ⑤ ⑥   BM #4 ① ② ③ ④ ⑤ ⑥

BM Notes

Do you need to call your doctor?   YES   NO

151

◯Ɔ **Breakfast** _____

◉ **Snack** _____

▢ **Lunch** _____

◉ **Snack** _____

🐑 **Dinner** _____

▭▭ **Exercise** _____ 🕐 **Time Spent Exercising** _____

✅ **What is one good thing that happened today?**

_____

📌 **What can you do to improve tomorrow?**

_____

📋 **Personal Journal / Notes** (write something about your day or personal thoughts)

_____

_____

_____

_____

_____

_____

Did you know?: Gallstones are more common in people with IBD due to the inability to properly absorb bile salts. The most common symptoms of gallstones are pain the lower or upper right hand part of the belly which can also migrate to the right upper back area.

31 Date _____

DAY 077

Temperature _____   **Weight** _____

Medications Taken Today

1 _____   2 _____   3 _____

Pain (Circle most painful moment)

0 — 1 — 2 — 3 — 4 — 5 — 6 — 7 — 8 — 9 — 10
GOOD   BAD

Types of Pain (circle all that apply)

| DULL | THROBBING | SHARP | CRAMPING |

How long did the pain last? (circle the longest time)

0 1 2 3 4 5 6 7 8 9 10 11 12 13 14 15 16 17 18 19 20 [More +]
Minutes

How many times have you experienced pain today? _____

Sickness Symptoms (cough, sweats, feel cold, loss of appetite)

Bowel Movements (bowel movement scale: 1 = Loose // 6 = Hard)

BM #1 ① ② ③ ④ ⑤ ⑥   BM #3 ① ② ③ ④ ⑤ ⑥
BM #2 ① ② ③ ④ ⑤ ⑥   BM #4 ① ② ③ ④ ⑤ ⑥

BM Notes _____

Do you need to call your doctor?   YES   NO

Breakfast

Snack

Lunch

Snack

Dinner

Exercise _____   Time Spent Exercising _____

✅ **What is one good thing that happened today?**

+1 **What can you do to improve tomorrow?**

📋 **Personal Journal / Notes** (write something about your day or personal thoughts)

31 Date _____

DAY 078

Temperature _____   **Weight** _____

Medications Taken Today

1 _____   2 _____   3 _____

Pain (Circle most painful moment)

0 1 2 3 4 5 6 7 8 9 **10**

GOOD   BAD

Types of Pain (circle all that apply)

DULL | THROBBING | SHARP | CRAMPING

How long did the pain last? (circle the longest time)

0 1 2 3 4 5 6 7 8 9 10 11 12 13 14 15 16 17 18 19 20 [More +]

Minutes

How many times have you experienced pain today? _____

Sickness Symptoms (cough, sweats, feel cold, loss of appetite)

_____

Bowel Movements (bowel movement scale: 1 = Loose // 6 = Hard)

BM #1 ① ② ③ 4 5 6   BM #3 ① ② ③ 4 5 6

BM #2 ① ② ③ 4 5 6   BM #4 ① ② ③ 4 5 6

BM Notes _____

Do you need to call your doctor?   YES   NO

◯⃝ **Breakfast** ▸_____

_____

◉ **Snack**   ▸_____

_____

☐ **Lunch**   ▸_____

_____

◉ **Snack**   ▸_____

_____

🍗 **Dinner**   ▸_____

_____

☷ **Exercise** ▸_____ ⏱ **Time Spent Exercising** ▸_____

✔ **What is one good thing that happened today?**

▸_____

◀1 **What can you do to improve tomorrow?**

▸_____

▤ **Personal Journal / Notes** (write something about your day or personal thoughts)

▸_____

_____

_____

_____

_____

_____

_____

The Mayo Clinic recommends 3 liters of water per day for men, and 2.2 liters per day for women. Tip: Find a water bottle that holds roughly 1 liter of water and drink 1 bottle in the morning, 1 bottle in the afternoon, and 1 bottle at night.

📅 Date ⟍_____

DAY 079

🌡 Temperature ⟍_____   👁 Weight ⟍_____

💊 Medications Taken Today

1 ⟍_____   2 ⟍_____   3 ⟍_____

Pain (Circle most painful moment)

(0) — (1) — (2) — (3) — (4) — (5) — (6) — (7) — (8) — (9) — (10)

GOOD   BAD

Types of Pain (circle all that apply)

DULL | **THROBBING** | **SHARP** | **CRAMPING**

How long did the pain last? (circle the longest time)

0 1 2 3 4 5 6 7 8 9 10 11 12 13 14 15 16 17 18 19 20 [More +]

Minutes

How many times have you experienced pain today? ⟍_____

⚡ Sickness Symptoms (cough, sweats, feel cold, loss of appetite)

_____

Bowel Movements (bowel movement scale: 1 = Loose // 6 = Hard)

BM #1 ❶ ❷ ❸ 4 5 6   BM #3 ❶ ❷ ❸ 4 5 6

BM #2 ❶ ❷ ❸ 4 5 6   BM #4 ❶ ❷ ❸ 4 5 6

BM Notes ⟍_____

🩺 Do you need to call your doctor? | YES | | NO |

157

◯◯ Breakfast _____

_____

◯ Snack _____

_____

▢ Lunch _____

_____

◯ Snack _____

_____

◯◯ Dinner _____

_____

◻◻ Exercise _____ ⏱ Time Spent Exercising _____

✔ What is one good thing that happened today?

_____

+1 What can you do to improve tomorrow?

_____

▤ Personal Journal / Notes (write something about your day or personal thoughts)

_____

_____

_____

_____

_____

_____

_____

_____

Did you know?: Most doctors agree that fast food isn't necessarily all bad for IBD patients. However, try to choose healthy options off the menu and avoid high fat foods, which can aggravate symptoms.

Date _____

DAY 080

Temperature _____   **Weight** _____

Medications Taken Today

1 _____   2 _____   3 _____

Pain (Circle most painful moment)

0 — 1 — 2 — 3 — 4 — 5 — 6 — 7 — 8 — 9 — 10
GOOD   BAD

Types of Pain (circle all that apply)

| DULL | THROBBING | SHARP | CRAMPING |

How long did the pain last? (circle the longest time)

0 1 2 3 4 5 6 7 8 9 10 11 12 13 14 15 16 17 18 19 20 [More +]
Minutes

How many times have you experienced pain today? _____

Sickness Symptoms (cough, sweats, feel cold, loss of appetite)

Bowel Movements (bowel movement scale: 1 = Loose // 6 = Hard)

BM #1 ① ② ③ ④ ⑤ ⑥   BM #3 ① ② ③ ④ ⑤ ⑥
BM #2 ① ② ③ ④ ⑤ ⑥   BM #4 ① ② ③ ④ ⑤ ⑥

BM Notes _____

Do you need to call your doctor?   YES   NO

159

○‿‿ Breakfast ▸_____

◉ Snack ▸_____

▢ Lunch ▸_____

◎ Snack ▸_____

🐑 Dinner ▸_____

O⊷O Exercise ▸_____ 🕐 Time Spent Exercising ▸_____

✅ What is one good thing that happened today?

▸_____

+1 What can you do to improve tomorrow?

▸_____

📋 Personal Journal / Notes (write something about your day or personal thoughts)

▸_____

_____

_____

_____

_____

_____

_____

📅 **Date** _____

DAY 081

🌡 **Temperature** _____ 👁 **Weight** _____

💊 **Medications Taken Today**

1 _____ 2 _____ 3 _____

Pain (Circle most painful moment)

0 1 2 3 4 5 6 7 8 9 10

GOOD   BAD

Types of Pain (circle all that apply)

| DULL | THROBBING | SHARP | CRAMPING |

How long did the pain last? (circle the longest time)

0 1 2 3 4 5 6 7 8 9 10 11 12 13 14 15 16 17 18 19 20 [More +]

Minutes

How many times have you experienced pain today? _____

⚡ **Sickness Symptoms** (cough, sweats, feel cold, loss of appetite)

_____

Bowel Movements (bowel movement scale: 1 = Loose // 6 = Hard)

BM #1 ① ② ③ ④ ⑤ ⑥   BM #3 ① ② ③ ④ ⑤ ⑥

BM #2 ① ② ③ ④ ⑤ ⑥   BM #4 ① ② ③ ④ ⑤ ⑥

BM Notes _____

🩺 **Do you need to call your doctor?**   YES   NO

161

◐ Breakfast ▸_____
_____

◉ Snack ▸_____
_____

▢ Lunch ▸_____
_____

◉ Snack ▸_____
_____

🐑 Dinner ▸_____
_____

▭ Exercise ▸_____ ⏱ Time Spent Exercising ▸_____

✔ **What is one good thing that happened today?**

▸_____

➕1 **What can you do to improve tomorrow?**

▸_____

▤ **Personal Journal / Notes** (write something about your day or personal thoughts)

▸_____
_____
_____
_____
_____
_____
_____

Tip: Lean proteins like chicken, fish and seafood are much more easily digestible than proteins from beef or pork, and they can be cooked almost any way you want.

Date _____

DAY 082

Temperature _____ **Weight** _____

Medications Taken Today

1 _____ 2 _____ 3 _____

Pain (Circle most painful moment)

0 — 1 — 2 — 3 — 4 — 5 — 6 — 7 — 8 — 9 — 10
GOOD   BAD

Types of Pain (circle all that apply)

| DULL | THROBBING | SHARP | CRAMPING |

How long did the pain last? (circle the longest time)

0 1 2 3 4 5 6 7 8 9 10 11 12 13 14 15 16 17 18 19 20 [More +]
Minutes

How many times have you experienced pain today? _____

Sickness Symptoms (cough, sweats, feel cold, loss of appetite)

Bowel Movements (bowel movement scale: 1 = Loose // 6 = Hard)

BM #1 ① ② ③ ④ ⑤ ⑥   BM #3 ① ② ③ ④ ⑤ ⑥

BM #2 ① ② ③ ④ ⑤ ⑥   BM #4 ① ② ③ ④ ⑤ ⑥

BM Notes _____

Do you need to call your doctor? YES   NO

163

⬭ Breakfast ▸_____

_____

◉ Snack ▸_____

_____

▢ Lunch ▸_____

_____

◉ Snack ▸_____

_____

🍗 Dinner ▸_____

_____

▭ Exercise ▸_____ ⏱ Time Spent Exercising ▸_____

✅ **What is one good thing that happened today?**

▸_____

📌 **What can you do to improve tomorrow?**

▸_____

📋 **Personal Journal / Notes** (write something about your day or personal thoughts)

▸_____

_____

_____

_____

_____

_____

_____

Date _____

DAY 083

Temperature _____   **Weight** _____

Medications Taken Today

1 _____   2 _____   3 _____

Pain (Circle most painful moment)

(0) (1) (2) (3) (4) (5) (6) (7) (8) (9) **(10)**

GOOD   BAD

Types of Pain (circle all that apply)

| DULL | THROBBING | SHARP | CRAMPING |

How long did the pain last? (circle the longest time)

0 1 2 3 4 5 6 7 8 9 10 11 12 13 14 15 16 17 18 19 20 [More +]

Minutes

How many times have you experienced pain today? _____

Sickness Symptoms (cough, sweats, feel cold, loss of appetite)

Bowel Movements (bowel movement scale: 1 = Loose // 6 = Hard)

BM #1 ① ② ③ ④ ⑤ ⑥   BM #3 ① ② ③ ④ ⑤ ⑥

BM #2 ① ② ③ ④ ⑤ ⑥   BM #4 ① ② ③ ④ ⑤ ⑥

BM Notes _____

Do you need to call your doctor?   [YES]   [NO]

165

◐ **Breakfast** _____

_____

◉ **Snack** _____

_____

⬜ **Lunch** _____

_____

◉ **Snack** _____

_____

🍗 **Dinner** _____

_____

▢–▢ **Exercise** _____ 🕐 **Time Spent Exercising** _____

✅ **What is one good thing that happened today?**

_____

+1 **What can you do to improve tomorrow?**

_____

▤ **Personal Journal / Notes** (write something about your day or personal thoughts)

_____

_____

_____

_____

_____

_____

_____

Did you know?: Protein is your body's main "repair" material. Try to incorporate at least two main sources of protein into your daily diet to help your body help itself.

Date _____

DAY 084

Temperature _____   **Weight** _____

Medications Taken Today

1 _____   2 _____   3 _____

Pain (Circle most painful moment)

⓪ ① ② ③ ④ ⑤ ⑥ ⑦ ⑧ ⑨ ⑩
GOOD   BAD

Types of Pain (circle all that apply)

| DULL | THROBBING | SHARP | CRAMPING |

How long did the pain last? (circle the longest time)

0 1 2 3 4 5 6 7 8 9 10 11 12 13 14 15 16 17 18 19 20 More +
Minutes

How many times have you experienced pain today? _____

Sickness Symptoms (cough, sweats, feel cold, loss of appetite)

Bowel Movements (bowel movement scale: 1 = Loose // 6 = Hard)

BM #1 ❶ ❷ ❸ ❹ ❺ ❻   BM #3 ❶ ❷ ❸ ❹ ❺ ❻

BM #2 ❶ ❷ ❸ ❹ ❺ ❻   BM #4 ❶ ❷ ❸ ❹ ❺ ❻

BM Notes _____

Do you need to call your doctor?   YES   NO

◯ **Breakfast** _____

_____

◉ **Snack** _____

_____

▢ **Lunch** _____

_____

◉ **Snack** _____

_____

🐓 **Dinner** _____

_____

◻ **Exercise** _____ ⏱ **Time Spent Exercising** _____

✔ **What is one good thing that happened today?**

_____

⁺❶ **What can you do to improve tomorrow?**

_____

▤ **Personal Journal / Notes** (write something about your day or personal thoughts)

_____

_____

_____

_____

_____

_____

_____

Did you know?: Night sweats are a good clue as to whether or not your condition is under control. If you are commonly experiencing night sweats, it probably isn't. Let your doctor know if you are experiencing common occurrences of night sweats.

📅 **Date** _____

DAY 085

🌡 **Temperature** _____   👁 **Weight** _____

💊 **Medications Taken Today**

1 _____ 2 _____ 3 _____

Pain (Circle most painful moment)

(0) (1) (2) (3) (4) (5) (6) (7) (8) (9) (10)

GOOD   BAD

Types of Pain (circle all that apply)

| DULL | THROBBING | SHARP | CRAMPING |

How long did the pain last? (circle the longest time)

0 1 2 3 4 5 6 7 8 9 10 11 12 13 14 15 16 17 18 19 20 [More +]

Minutes

How many times have you experienced pain today? _____

⚡ **Sickness Symptoms** (cough, sweats, feel cold, loss of appetite)

_____

Bowel Movements (bowel movement scale: 1 = Loose // 6 = Hard)

BM #1 ❶ ❷ ❸ 4 5 6   BM #3 ❶ ❷ 3 4 5 6

BM #2 ❶ ❷ ❸ 4 5 6   BM #4 ❶ ❷ 3 4 5 6

BM Notes _____

🩺 **Do you need to call your doctor?** | YES | | NO |

169

◯▷ Breakfast ▸_____

◯ Snack ▸_____

◻ Lunch ▸_____

◯ Snack ▸_____

🐑 Dinner ▸_____

▭▭ Exercise ▸_____ 🕐 Time Spent Exercising ▸_____

✅ **What is one good thing that happened today?**

▸_____

📌 **What can you do to improve tomorrow?**

▸_____

📋 **Personal Journal / Notes** (write something about your day or personal thoughts)

▸_____

_____

_____

_____

_____

_____

_____

Tip: Eggs are a great source of easily digestible protein and can help make a great meal, even during a flare.

📅 **Date** _____

DAY 086

🌡️ **Temperature** _____ 👁️ **Weight** _____

💊 **Medications Taken Today**

1 _____ 2 _____ 3 _____

Pain (Circle most painful moment)

0 — 1 — 2 — 3 — 4 — 5 — 6 — 7 — 8 — 9 — **10**
GOOD .... BAD

Types of Pain (circle all that apply)

| DULL | THROBBING | SHARP | CRAMPING |

How long did the pain last? (circle the longest time)

0 1 2 3 4 5 6 7 8 9 10 11 12 13 14 15 16 17 18 19 20 [More +]
Minutes

How many times have you experienced pain today? _____

⚡ **Sickness Symptoms** (cough, sweats, feel cold, loss of appetite)

_____

⚱️ **Bowel Movements** (bowel movement scale: 1 = Loose // 6 = Hard)

BM #1 ① ② 3 4 5 6   BM #3 ① ② 3 4 5 6

BM #2 ① ② 3 4 5 6   BM #4 ① ② 3 4 5 6

BM Notes _____

🩺 **Do you need to call your doctor?** | YES | | NO |

◯ **Breakfast** ▄_____

_____

◉ **Snack** ▄_____

_____

▢ **Lunch** ▄_____

_____

◉ **Snack** ▄_____

_____

🎧 **Dinner** ▄_____

_____

〇〇 **Exercise** ▄_____ ◷ **Time Spent Exercising** ▄_____

✔ **What is one good thing that happened today?**

▄_____

+1 **What can you do to improve tomorrow?**

▄_____

▤ **Personal Journal / Notes** (write something about your day or personal thoughts)

▄_____

_____

_____

_____

_____

_____

_____

📅 **Date** _____

DAY 087

🌡 **Temperature** _____   👁 **Weight** _____

💊 **Medications Taken Today**

1 _____   2 _____   3 _____

Pain (Circle most painful moment)

(0) (1) (2) (3) (4) (5) (6) (7) (8) (9) (10)

GOOD   BAD

Types of Pain (circle all that apply)

| DULL | THROBBING | SHARP | CRAMPING |

How long did the pain last? (circle the longest time)

0 1 2 3 4 5 6 7 8 9 10 11 12 13 14 15 16 17 18 19 20 [More +]

Minutes

How many times have you experienced pain today? _____

⚡ **Sickness Symptoms** (cough, sweats, feel cold, loss of appetite)

_____

Bowel Movements (bowel movement scale: 1 = Loose // 6 = Hard)

BM #1 **1** **2** **3** **4** **5** **6**   BM #3 **1** **2** **3** **4** **5** **6**

BM #2 **1** **2** **3** **4** **5** **6**   BM #4 **1** **2** **3** **4** **5** **6**

BM Notes _____

🩺 **Do you need to call your doctor?** | YES | | NO |

◐ **Breakfast** _____

◉ **Snack** _____

◻ **Lunch** _____

◉ **Snack** _____

🐑 **Dinner** _____

○○ **Exercise** _____ ⊘ **Time Spent Exercising** _____

✔ **What is one good thing that happened today?**

_____

◀ **What can you do to improve tomorrow?**

_____

▤ **Personal Journal / Notes** (write something about your day or personal thoughts)

_____

_____

_____

_____

_____

_____

_____

> **Tip:** When planning to travel for an extended time (more than 1 week), notify your doctor and ask him or her to recommend a doctor in the location to which you will be traveling. This can help put your mind at ease, and it is a good safety measure.

Date _____

DAY 088

Temperature _____   **Weight** _____

Medications Taken Today

1 _____   2 _____   3 _____

Pain (Circle most painful moment)

(0) (1) (2) (3) (4) (5) (6) (7) (8) (9) (10)

GOOD   BAD

Types of Pain (circle all that apply)

| DULL | THROBBING | SHARP | CRAMPING |

How long did the pain last? (circle the longest time)

0 1 2 3 4 5 6 7 8 9 10 11 12 13 14 15 16 17 18 19 20 [More +]

Minutes

How many times have you experienced pain today? _____

Sickness Symptoms (cough, sweats, feel cold, loss of appetite)

_____

Bowel Movements (bowel movement scale: 1 = Loose // 6 = Hard)

BM #1 ① ② ③ ④ ⑤ ⑥   BM #3 ① ② ③ ④ ⑤ ⑥

BM #2 ① ② ③ ④ ⑤ ⑥   BM #4 ① ② ③ ④ ⑤ ⑥

BM Notes _____

Do you need to call your doctor?   [YES]   [NO]

175

○ Breakfast

○ Snack

○ Lunch

○ Snack

○ Dinner

○ Exercise _____ ○ Time Spent Exercising _____

✅ What is one good thing that happened today?

📌 What can you do to improve tomorrow?

📋 Personal Journal / Notes (write something about your day or personal thoughts)

Tip: To avoid aggravating symptoms, avoid eating at least 2 hours before going to bed. If that's not possible, go for a 20-minute walk before bed to aid your body's digestion.

📅 Date _____

DAY 089

🌡️ Temperature _____   **⚖️ Weight** _____

💊 Medications Taken Today

1 _____   2 _____   3 _____

Pain (Circle most painful moment)

0 — 1 — 2 — 3 — 4 — 5 — 6 — 7 — 8 — 9 — **10**
GOOD   BAD

Types of Pain (circle all that apply)

| DULL | THROBBING | SHARP | CRAMPING |

How long did the pain last? (circle the longest time)

0 1 2 3 4 5 6 7 8 9 10 11 12 13 14 15 16 17 18 19 20 [More +]
Minutes

How many times have you experienced pain today? _____

⚡ Sickness Symptoms (cough, sweats, feel cold, loss of appetite)

_____

Bowel Movements (bowel movement scale: 1 = Loose // 6 = Hard)

BM #1 ① ② ③ ④ ⑤ ⑥   BM #3 ① ② ③ ④ ⑤ ⑥

BM #2 ① ② ③ ④ ⑤ ⑥   BM #4 ① ② ③ ④ ⑤ ⑥

BM Notes _____

🩺 Do you need to call your doctor? | YES | | NO |

177

◯ **Breakfast** _____

_____

◯ **Snack** _____

_____

▢ **Lunch** _____

_____

◯ **Snack** _____

_____

Dinner _____

_____

Exercise _____   ◯ **Time Spent Exercising** _____

✔ **What is one good thing that happened today?**

_____

What can you do to improve tomorrow?

_____

▤ **Personal Journal / Notes** (write something about your day or personal thoughts)

_____

_____

_____

_____

_____

_____

_____

Tip: It is usually a good idea to avoid foods that are highly acidic, such as 100 percent juice drinks, acid tomato sauces, coffee and sodas. The acid in these drinks can irritate the bowels and exacerbate symptoms.

DAY 090

📅 Date _____

🌡 Temperature _____ 🌡 Weight _____

💊 **Medications Taken Today**

1 _____ 2 _____ 3 _____

Pain (Circle most painful moment)

0 — 1 — 2 — 3 — 4 — 5 — 6 — 7 — 8 — 9 — **10**
GOOD   BAD

Types of Pain (circle all that apply)

| DULL | THROBBING | SHARP | CRAMPING |

How long did the pain last? (circle the longest time)

0 1 2 3 4 5 6 7 8 9 10 11 12 13 14 15 16 17 18 19 20 [More +]
Minutes

How many times have you experienced pain today? _____

⚡ **Sickness Symptoms** (cough, sweats, feel cold, loss of appetite)

_____

Bowel Movements (bowel movement scale: 1 = Loose // 6 = Hard)

BM #1 **1** **2** 3 4 5 6   BM #3 **1** 2 3 4 5 6
BM #2 **1** **2** 3 4 5 6   BM #4 **1** **2** 3 4 5 6

BM Notes _____

🩺 **Do you need to call your doctor?**   YES   NO

◯▷ **Breakfast** ⬏_____

⊙ **Snack** ⬏_____

◻ **Lunch** ⬏_____

⊙ **Snack** ⬏_____

🐑 **Dinner** ⬏_____

O-O **Exercise** ⬏_____   ⊘ **Time Spent Exercising** ⬏_____

✅ **What is one good thing that happened today?**

⬏_____

+1 **What can you do to improve tomorrow?**

⬏_____

▤ **Personal Journal / Notes** (write something about your day or personal thoughts)

⬏_____

_____

_____

_____

_____

_____

_____

Did you know?: Peanut butter and other nut butters are a great source of protein and can help if you have a craving for nuts. Make sure you only choose smooth nut butters, as others are more difficult to digest.

📅 Date _____

DAY 091

🌡 Temperature _____   **👁 Weight** _____

💊 Medications Taken Today

1 _____   2 _____   3 _____

Pain (Circle most painful moment)

⓪ ① ② ③ ④ ⑤ ⑥ ⑦ ⑧ ⑨ ⑩

GOOD   BAD

Types of Pain (circle all that apply)

| DULL | THROBBING | SHARP | CRAMPING |

How long did the pain last? (circle the longest time)

0 1 2 3 4 5 6 7 8 9 10 11 12 13 14 15 16 17 18 19 20 [More +]

Minutes

How many times have you experienced pain today? _____

⚡ Sickness Symptoms (cough, sweats, feel cold, loss of appetite)

_____

Bowel Movements (bowel movement scale: 1 = Loose // 6 = Hard)

BM #1 ❶ ❷ ❸ 4 5 6   BM #3 ❶ ❷ 3 4 5 6

BM #2 ❶ ❷ ❸ ❹ 5 6   BM #4 ❶ ❷ 3 4 5 6

BM Notes _____

🩺 Do you need to call your doctor? | YES | | NO |

○D **Breakfast** ▸_____

⊙ **Snack** ▸_____

▢ **Lunch** ▸_____

⊙ **Snack** ▸_____

🍗 **Dinner** ▸_____

⊶ **Exercise** ▸_____ 🕐 **Time Spent Exercising** ▸_____

✔ **What is one good thing that happened today?**

▸_____

📌 **What can you do to improve tomorrow?**

▸_____

▤ **Personal Journal / Notes** (write something about your day or personal thoughts)

▸_____

_____

_____

_____

_____

_____

_____

> Tip: Antidiarrheal drugs can be beneficial for IBD patients; however, it is important to not become dependent or overuse them. Overuse can lead to an impacted colon, especially during a flare.

Date _____

Temperature _____   **Weight** _____

Medications Taken Today

1 _____   2 _____   3 _____

Pain (Circle most painful moment)

0 — 1 — 2 — 3 — 4 — 5 — 6 — **7** — 8 — 9 — **10**

GOOD   BAD

Types of Pain (circle all that apply)

| DULL | THROBBING | SHARP | CRAMPING |

How long did the pain last? (circle the longest time)

0 1 2 3 4 5 6 7 8 9 10 11 12 13 14 15 16 17 18 19 20 [More +]

Minutes

How many times have you experienced pain today? _____

Sickness Symptoms (cough, sweats, feel cold, loss of appetite)

Bowel Movements (bowel movement scale: 1 = Loose // 6 = Hard)

BM #1 **1** **2** 3 4 5 6   BM #3 **1** **2** 3 4 5 6

BM #2 **1** **2** 3 4 5 6   BM #4 **1** **2** 3 4 5 6

BM Notes _____

Do you need to call your doctor?   YES   NO

○ Breakfast _____

○ Snack _____

□ Lunch _____

○ Snack _____

○ Dinner _____

○○ Exercise _____ ○ Time Spent Exercising _____

✔ **What is one good thing that happened today?**

_____

+1 **What can you do to improve tomorrow?**

_____

▤ **Personal Journal / Notes** (write something about your day or personal thoughts)

_____

_____

_____

_____

_____

_____

_____

Famous People with IBD: Al Geiberger, a former professional American golfer who has won 11 PGA Tour tournaments.

Date _____

DAY 093

Temperature _____   **Weight** _____

Medications Taken Today

1 _____   2 _____   3 _____

Pain (Circle most painful moment)

0 — 1 — 2 — 3 — 4 — 5 — 6 — 7 — 8 — 9 — 10
GOOD   BAD

Types of Pain (circle all that apply)

| DULL | THROBBING | SHARP | CRAMPING |

How long did the pain last? (circle the longest time)

0 1 2 3 4 5 6 7 8 9 10 11 12 13 14 15 16 17 18 19 20 [More +]
Minutes

How many times have you experienced pain today? _____

Sickness Symptoms (cough, sweats, feel cold, loss of appetite)

Bowel Movements (bowel movement scale: 1 = Loose // 6 = Hard)

BM #1 ① ② ③ ④ ⑤ ⑥   BM #3 ① ② ③ ④ ⑤ ⑥

BM #2 ① ② ③ ④ ⑤ ⑥   BM #4 ① ② ③ ④ ⑤ ⑥

BM Notes _____

Do you need to call your doctor? | YES | | NO |

185

○ **Breakfast** _____

_____

○ **Snack** _____

_____

○ **Lunch** _____

_____

○ **Snack** _____

_____

○ **Dinner** _____

_____

○ **Exercise** _____   ○ **Time Spent Exercising** _____

✓ **What is one good thing that happened today?**

_____

◀ **What can you do to improve tomorrow?**

_____

▤ **Personal Journal / Notes** (write something about your day or personal thoughts)

_____

_____

_____

_____

_____

_____

_____

Tip: Stick to a set daily routine in order to reduce stress and overcome the "blah" days. Keep a planner or set activities in your phone.

📅 Date _____

DAY 094

🌡 Temperature _____   👁 Weight _____

💊 **Medications Taken Today**

1 _____   2 _____   3 _____

Pain (Circle most painful moment)

0 — 1 — 2 — 3 — 4 — 5 — 6 — 7 — 8 — 9 — 10
GOOD   BAD

Types of Pain (circle all that apply)

| DULL | THROBBING | SHARP | CRAMPING |

How long did the pain last? (circle the longest time)

0 1 2 3 4 5 6 7 8 9 10 11 12 13 14 15 16 17 18 19 20 [More +]
Minutes

How many times have you experienced pain today? _____

⚡ **Sickness Symptoms** (cough, sweats, feel cold, loss of appetite)

_____

Bowel Movements (bowel movement scale: 1 = Loose // 6 = Hard)

BM #1 ① ② ③ ④ ⑤ ⑥   BM #3 ① ② ③ ④ ⑤ ⑥
BM #2 ① ② ③ ④ ⑤ ⑥   BM #4 ① ② ③ ④ ⑤ ⑥

BM Notes _____

🩺 **Do you need to call your doctor?**   [YES]   [NO]

187

⚬ **Breakfast** ➤ _____

⊚ **Snack** ➤ _____

⬚ **Lunch** ➤ _____

⊚ **Snack** ➤ _____

🍗 **Dinner** ➤ _____

🏋 **Exercise** ➤ _____ 🕐 **Time Spent Exercising** ➤ _____

✓ **What is one good thing that happened today?**

➤ _____

+1 **What can you do to improve tomorrow?**

➤ _____

📋 **Personal Journal / Notes** (write something about your day or personal thoughts)

➤ _____

_____

_____

_____

_____

_____

📅 **Date** _____

DAY 095

🌡 **Temperature** _____   👁 **Weight** _____

💊 **Medications Taken Today**

1 _____   2 _____   3 _____

Pain (Circle most painful moment)

⓪ ① ② ③ ④ ⑤ ⑥ ⑦ ⑧ ⑨ ⑩
GOOD   BAD

Types of Pain (circle all that apply)

| DULL | THROBBING | SHARP | CRAMPING |

How long did the pain last? (circle the longest time)

0 1 2 3 4 5 6 7 8 9 10 11 12 13 14 15 16 17 18 19 20 [More +]
Minutes

How many times have you experienced pain today? _____

⚡ **Sickness Symptoms** (cough, sweats, feel cold, loss of appetite)

_____

Bowel Movements (bowel movement scale: 1 = Loose // 6 = Hard)

BM #1 ❶ ❷ ❸ ❹ ❺ ❻   BM #3 ❶ ❷ ❸ ❹ ❺ ❻

BM #2 ❶ ❷ ❸ ❹ ❺ ❻   BM #4 ❶ ❷ ❸ ❹ ❺ ❻

BM Notes _____

🩺 **Do you need to call your doctor?** | YES | | NO |

189

⬭ **Breakfast** ▸_____

⊙ **Snack** ▸_____

⬜ **Lunch** ▸_____

⊙ **Snack** ▸_____

🐑 **Dinner** ▸_____

⊟ **Exercise** ▸_____ 🕐 **Time Spent Exercising** ▸_____

✅ **What is one good thing that happened today?**

▸_____

📌 **What can you do to improve tomorrow?**

▸_____

📋 **Personal Journal / Notes** (write something about your day or personal thoughts)

▸_____

_____

_____

_____

_____

_____

_____

📅 **Date** _____

DAY 096

🌡 **Temperature** _____   👁 **Weight** _____

💊 **Medications Taken Today**

1 _____   2 _____   3 _____

🩹 **Pain** (Circle most painful moment)

0 — 1 — 2 — 3 — 4 — 5 — 6 — 7 — 8 — 9 — **10**
GOOD   BAD

Types of Pain (circle all that apply)

| DULL | THROBBING | SHARP | CRAMPING |

How long did the pain last? (circle the longest time)

0 1 2 3 4 5 6 7 8 9 10 11 12 13 14 15 16 17 18 19 20 [More +]
Minutes

How many times have you experienced pain today? _____

⚡ **Sickness Symptoms** (cough, sweats, feel cold, loss of appetite)

_____

🏺 **Bowel Movements** (bowel movement scale: 1 = Loose // 6 = Hard)

BM #1 ① ② ③ ④ ⑤ ⑥   BM #3 ① ② ③ ④ ⑤ ⑥

BM #2 ① ② ③ ④ ⑤ ⑥   BM #4 ① ② ③ ④ ⑤ ⑥

BM Notes _____

🩺 **Do you need to call your doctor?** | YES | | NO |

191

ᗺ Breakfast ⬤_____

_____

◉ Snack ⬤_____

_____

▢ Lunch ⬤_____

_____

◉ Snack ⬤_____

_____

🐑 Dinner ⬤_____

_____

O═O Exercise ⬤_____ ⏱ Time Spent Exercising ⬤_____

✔ **What is one good thing that happened today?**

⬤_____

📌 **What can you do to improve tomorrow?**

⬤_____

📄 **Personal Journal / Notes** (write something about your day or personal thoughts)

⬤_____

_____

_____

_____

_____

_____

_____

Tip: If you have children or are having a hard time explaining your disease to someone, try drawing a diagram to explain how it affects you. This also helps if you have a child with IBD and need to explain how taking their medication can help them.

📅 **Date** _____

DAY 097

🌡️ **Temperature** _____   ⚖️ **Weight** _____

💊 **Medications Taken Today**

1 _____   2 _____   3 _____

Pain (Circle most painful moment)

0 — 1 — 2 — 3 — 4 — 5 — 6 — 7 — 8 — 9 — **10**
GOOD   BAD

Types of Pain (circle all that apply)

| DULL | THROBBING | SHARP | CRAMPING |

How long did the pain last? (circle the longest time)

0 1 2 3 4 5 6 7 8 9 10 11 12 13 14 15 16 17 18 19 20 [More +]
Minutes

How many times have you experienced pain today? _____

⚡ **Sickness Symptoms** (cough, sweats, feel cold, loss of appetite)

_____

🏺 **Bowel Movements** (bowel movement scale: 1 = Loose // 6 = Hard)

BM #1 **1** 2 3 4 5 6   BM #3 **1** **2** 3 4 5 6

BM #2 **1** **2** 3 4 5 6   BM #4 **1** **2** 3 4 5 6

BM Notes _____

🩺 **Do you need to call your doctor?**   [YES]   [NO]

Breakfast ▸_____

_____

Snack ▸_____

_____

Lunch ▸_____

_____

Snack ▸_____

_____

Dinner ▸_____

_____

Exercise ▸_____   Time Spent Exercising ▸_____

✔ **What is one good thing that happened today?**

▸_____

📌 **What can you do to improve tomorrow?**

▸_____

▤ **Personal Journal / Notes** (write something about your day or personal thoughts)

▸_____

_____

_____

_____

_____

_____

_____

31 Date _____

DAY 098

Temperature _____ **Weight** _____

Medications Taken Today

1 _____ 2 _____ 3 _____

Pain (Circle most painful moment)

0 1 2 3 4 5 6 7 8 9 **10**

GOOD   BAD

Types of Pain (circle all that apply)

| DULL | THROBBING | SHARP | CRAMPING |

How long did the pain last? (circle the longest time)

0 1 2 3 4 5 6 7 8 9 10 11 12 13 14 15 16 17 18 19 20 [More +]

Minutes

How many times have you experienced pain today? _____

Sickness Symptoms (cough, sweats, feel cold, loss of appetite)

_____

Bowel Movements (bowel movement scale: 1 = Loose // 6 = Hard)

BM #1 **1** **2** 3 4 5 6   BM #3 **1** 2 3 4 5 6

BM #2 **1** **2** 3 4 5 6   BM #4 **1** **2** 3 4 5 6

BM Notes _____

Do you need to call your doctor? | YES | | NO |

Breakfast _____

Snack _____

Lunch _____

Snack _____

Dinner _____

Exercise _____ Time Spent Exercising _____

What is one good thing that happened today?

_____

What can you do to improve tomorrow?

_____

Personal Journal / Notes (write something about your day or personal thoughts)

_____

_____

_____

_____

_____

_____

_____

Date ⬣_____

DAY 099

Temperature ⬣_____   👁 **Weight** ⬣_____

Medications Taken Today

1 ⬣_____   2 ⬣_____   3 ⬣_____

Pain (Circle most painful moment)

⓪ ① ② ③ ④ ⑤ ⑥ ⑦ ⑧ ⑨ ⑩

GOOD   BAD

Types of Pain (circle all that apply)

| DULL | THROBBING | SHARP | CRAMPING |

How long did the pain last? (circle the longest time)

0 1 2 3 4 5 6 7 8 9 10 11 12 13 14 15 16 17 18 19 20 [More +]

Minutes

How many times have you experienced pain today? ⬣_____

Sickness Symptoms (cough, sweats, feel cold, loss of appetite)

Bowel Movements (bowel movement scale: 1 = Loose // 6 = Hard)

BM #1 ① ② ③ ④ ⑤ ⑥   BM #3 ① ② ③ ④ ⑤ ⑥

BM #2 ① ② ③ ④ ⑤ ⑥   BM #4 ① ② ③ ④ ⑤ ⑥

BM Notes ⬣_____

Do you need to call your doctor?   YES   NO

◯ **Breakfast** _____

◉ **Snack** _____

▢ **Lunch** _____

◉ **Snack** _____

🐑 **Dinner** _____

□—□ **Exercise** _____ 🕐 **Time Spent Exercising** _____

✓ **What is one good thing that happened today?**

_____

+1 **What can you do to improve tomorrow?**

_____

▤ **Personal Journal / Notes** (write something about your day or personal thoughts)

_____

_____

_____

_____

_____

_____

Tip: If you're having a hard time feeling finished during a BM, try moving your upper body in a circular or figure-eight pattern while sitting upright. This should help to get anything left moving and ensure completion.

Date _____

DAY 100

Temperature _____   **Weight** _____

Medications Taken Today

1 _____   2 _____   3 _____

Pain (Circle most painful moment)

0 — 1 — 2 — 3 — 4 — 5 — 6 — 7 — 8 — 9 — **10**

GOOD   BAD

Types of Pain (circle all that apply)

| DULL | THROBBING | SHARP | CRAMPING |

How long did the pain last? (circle the longest time)

0 1 2 3 4 5 6 7 8 9 10 11 12 13 14 15 16 17 18 19 20 [More +]

Minutes

How many times have you experienced pain today? _____

Sickness Symptoms (cough, sweats, feel cold, loss of appetite)

Bowel Movements (bowel movement scale: 1 = Loose // 6 = Hard)

BM #1 **1** **2** 3 4 5 6   BM #3 **1** **2** 3 4 5 6

BM #2 **1** **2** 3 4 5 6   BM #4 **1** **2** 3 4 5 6

BM Notes _____

Do you need to call your doctor?   YES   NO

○ Breakfast _____

○ Snack _____

▢ Lunch _____

○ Snack _____

○ Dinner _____

○─○ Exercise _____ ○ Time Spent Exercising _____

✔ What is one good thing that happened today?

_____

+1 What can you do to improve tomorrow?

_____

▤ Personal Journal / Notes (write something about your day or personal thoughts)

_____

_____

_____

_____

_____

_____

_____

📅 **Date** ↳_____

DAY 101

🌡 **Temperature** ↳_____ ⚖ **Weight** ↳_____

💊 **Medications Taken Today**

1 ↳_____ 2 ↳_____ 3 ↳_____

Pain (Circle most painful moment)

⓿—①—②—③—④—⑤—⑥—⑦—⑧—⑨—⑩

GOOD   BAD

Types of Pain (circle all that apply)

| DULL | THROBBING | SHARP | CRAMPING |

How long did the pain last? (circle the longest time)

0 1 2 3 4 5 6 7 8 9 10 11 12 13 14 15 16 17 18 19 20 [More +]

Minutes

How many times have you experienced pain today? ↳_____

⚡ **Sickness Symptoms** (cough, sweats, feel cold, loss of appetite)

_____

Bowel Movements (bowel movement scale: 1 = Loose // 6 = Hard)

BM #1 ❶ ❷ ❸ ❹ ❺ ❻   BM #3 ❶ ❷ ❸ ❹ ❺ ❻

BM #2 ❶ ❷ ❸ ❹ ❺ ❻   BM #4 ❶ ❷ ❸ ❹ ❺ ❻

BM Notes ↳_____

🩺 **Do you need to call your doctor?**   [YES]   [NO]

◯ **Breakfast** _____

◉ **Snack** _____

▢ **Lunch** _____

◉ **Snack** _____

🐔 **Dinner** _____

O─O **Exercise** _____ 🕐 **Time Spent Exercising** _____

✅ **What is one good thing that happened today?**

_____

+1 **What can you do to improve tomorrow?**

_____

▤ **Personal Journal / Notes** (write something about your day or personal thoughts)

_____

_____

_____

_____

_____

_____

FOOD LOG

😊 **Foods To Enjoy**   😕 **Foods To avoid**

	Foods To Enjoy		Foods To avoid
1		1	
2		2	
3		3	
4		4	
5		5	
6		6	
7		7	
8		8	
9		9	
10		10	
11		11	
12		12	
13		13	
14		14	
15		15	
16		16	
17		17	
18		18	
19		19	
20		20	
21		21	
22		22	
23		23	
24		24	
25		25	

MEDICAL INFORMATION

My Medications & Supplements

1 _____

2 _____

3 _____

4 _____

5 _____

Recommended Vaccinations

- Flu Shot (1 time each year)
- Pneumonia Vaccine (1 time every 5 years)
- Shingles Vaccine (just once)

Questions For Doctor _____ (Fill this in)

1 _____
_____

Answer _____
_____

2 _____
_____

Answer _____
_____

3 _____
_____

Answer _____
_____

4 _____
_____

Answer _____
_____

FAMILY TREE

Mother's Family

Father's Family

Mother's Great-Grandmother

Mother's Great-Grandfather

Mother's Grandmother

Mother's Grandfather

Mother's Mother

Mother's Father

Father's Great-Grandmother

Father's Great-Grandfather

Father's Grandmother

Father's Grandfather

Father's Mother

Father's Father

Me

Knowing your family's genealogy of traits and diseases can help your doctor to assess certain risks and determine which medications may be best for you.

TIPS

1. Did you know?: Creating a detailed history of family members who have had any medical conditions can help your doctor to correctly asses medications that should be prescribed. Use the Family Tree example diagram in the back of this journal to map out any family members with any known medical conditions.
2. Tip: If you have a child with IBD, remember that it may be difficult for them to talk about some of their symptoms. Help them to find creative ways to stay on top of their disease by suggesting blogging, journaling, keeping a diary, finding a confidant, or any other means of recording or reporting their condition.
3. Did you know?: Lower back pain can be quite common for people with IBD and may come or go with symptoms. This may be because of arthritis caused by the IBD or kidney stones. Check with your doctor if you are experiencing lower back pain, especially if you experience it along with other symptoms.
4. Tip: Try an avocado—This fruit is full of good fats, B vitamins, vitamin E, and soluble, as well as insoluble fiber.
5. Famous People with IBD: Matt Light, a former American football offensive tackle for the New England Patriots.
6. Famous People with IBD: Ben Morrison, famous stand-up comedian and actor.
7. Tip: Try almond milk as an accompaniment to your morning breakfast. Almond milk is full of calcium, protein, and vitamin E and comes in a variety of flavors.
8. Did you know?: Red bumps, called erythema nodosum, can appear on the shin or ankles and are more common in women than men. For people with IBD, these commonly occur just before or during a flare.
9. Tip: In addition to brushing your teeth, use a mouthwash. Doing something as simple as this can help you to avoid infections.
10. Famous People with IBD: John F. Kennedy, the 35th president of the United States, also suffered from adrenal deficiency, osteoporosis, and multiple infections throughout his presidency.
11. Tip: Use the "Questions for Doctor_____" portion of this journal to keep a set of questions for your doctor for every visit. The more you ask, the more you will know and the better off you will be.
12. Did you know?: White rice is a great staple and fallback if you are experiencing symptoms. It is easy to digest and contains calories, which can help during flares.

13. Famous People with IBD: Cynthia McFadden, news correspondent for ABC News and co-anchor of Primetime and Nightline.
14. Tip: Avoid food with large indigestible fibers. If it looks like it won't digest, it probably won't. Some examples include corn, nuts, raw veggies, and raw fruits with skins or thick fibers. The good news is that many raw veggies and fruits can be cooked to make them easily digestible.
15. Tip: The more detail the better. It can be difficult to talk specifically about bowel movements, stool contents, pain, cramping, or other symptoms, but the more your doctor knows, the better he can treat you. Elaborate on every detail you know to be certain your doctor has a clear picture of your situation.
16. Tip: Try Boost or Ensure as a simple between-meal snack. It is pumped full of nutrients, minerals, and protein.
17. Famous People with IBD: Kevin Dineen, former NHL player and current hockey coach of the Florida Panthers.
18. Tip: Maintain a normal sleep schedule. Maintaining a simple schedule helps you to know when you may be experiencing an increase in symptoms and may help you to head off a flare.
19. Tip: Stay intimate. Don't shy away from intimacy because of symptoms: Let your partner know what feels good, such as kissing, hugging or just being together.
20. Tip: Ask your doctor to write down all instructions and details from your visit. Keeping these in chronological order can help future doctors' overview your treatment and past.
21. Did you know?: You don't have to avoid all fruits! Bananas, papaya, cantaloupe, and mango are all easily digestible fruits that are rich in vitamins and minerals, many of which can aid in the digestion of proteins.
22. Did you know?: Most doctors recommend that you only use Tylenol, or a similar generic, as an over-the-counter medicine to manage mild pain. This is because it is less harsh on your system.
23. Tip: Schedule something in your week to look forward to, whether it be movies with a friend or a public outing. Use this as motivational force if your week hasn't gone quite as planned.
24. Famous People with IBD: Anastacia, a widely popular American singer/songwriter.

25. Did you know?: Taking a calcium tablet along with your morning vitamins is recommended by many doctors. This is because some medications, specifically corticosteroids, can increase risk for osteoporosis, and in specific cases it may help to reduce chances of kidney stones.

26. Did you know?: Stress can affect the body hours after the stressful situation has passed. Muscles can remain flexed and taut, causing chain reactions throughout your body, including your gut. Try taking a walk or exercising directly after a stressful event to head off any symptoms.

27. Did You Know?: You are at high risk of dehydration during a flare. Drink water as much as possible to reduce symptoms and increase your body's ability to recover.

28. Famous People with IBD: Carrie Johnson, a former American Summer Olympics sprint canoer.

29. Tip: Use the "Foods to Enjoy" portion of this journal to keep a list of foods that you know work well for you and new foods you find work well. It also makes for a quick shopping list and easy reference for relatives or friends who want to know; "What can you eat?"

30. Did you know?: Many people with IBD do not handle fiber well. Try a low fiber diet for 1 week and see if you feel any different.

31. Tip: Oatmeal, which has soluble fiber, can be a great meal even during a flare. Soluble fiber passes more slowly through the digestive system and absorbs water, which can help with loose stools.

32. Tip: Don't forget to ask your doctor about getting your flu shot and pneumonia vaccine. These simple measures can help avoid some nasty downtime.

33. Tip: Have you noticed any foods that cause you discomfort or increased gas? If so, mark them down in the back of your journal under the Foods to Avoid page. If you are on the fence about a food option, use the 3-strikes rule and see if eating that food affects you similarly more than once.

34. Did you know?: Some IBD patients have claimed that taking Chlorella supplements can help to alleviate gas and decrease toxins in the body. As always, you should consult your doctor before taking any additional supplements or medications.

35. Famous People with IBD: Dynamo, an English magician best known for his documentary show, Dynamo.

36. Tip: When traveling, bring snacks you know will "sit well with" your system; map out bathroom stops and restaurants you know will work well for you.

37. Tip: If you have problems with an excess amount of gas, ask your doctor about taking simethicone. Taking this over-the-counter medication after meals can greatly reduce gas and odor.

38. Did you know?: Studies have not been able to definitively prove that Crohn's will be inherited following the normal Mendelian Inheritance guidelines (passing of a certain trait onto your children or the trait skipping a generation.) At best, they estimate there is a 1 in 5 chance of a child developing it if there is a family history of Crohn's.

39. Tip: Try using a blender or blend stick with steamed vegetables such as lentils, butternut squash, parsnips, pumpkin and carrots to make creamy vegetable soups. By blending them, you won't lose as many nutrients as you would boiling and mashing them, and you can still enjoy a healthy nutritious meal.

40. Famous People with IBD: Mary Ann Mobley, a former Miss America, actress, and television personality.

41. Famous People with IBD: Dwight D. Eisenhower, WWII general and 34th president of the United States.

42. Did you know?: Many people with IBD do not even realize when they are running a fever. Low grade fevers do not usually affect daily activities but are good indicators of how well your condition is under control. Check your temperature daily to see how you are doing.

43. Did you know?: Specific medications such as Prednisone and Sulfasalazine can deplete the body of nutrients or require you to intake additional nutrients or calories. Ask your doctor about any supplements or minerals you should be taking along with your medication.

44. Tip: If you are starting to feel under the weather or think maybe your gut just needs a rest, try a bland diet for one day. A bland diet can consist of limited amounts of fish, pureed veggies, pureed low acid fruits, crackers, plain bread, water, and anything else you have found to be very easily digestible.

45. Famous People with IBD: Frank Fritz, co-star on the History Channel series, American Pickers.

46. Tip: While cancer is a difficult subject to approach, it is not a subject that should be avoided with your doctor. Patients with IBD are at a greater risk for some forms of cancer and should be aware of early detection techniques.

47. Tip: People on corticosteroids should be evaluated by an eye doctor every 6 months for a routine eye examination. This is because corticosteroids increase the risk of eye inflammation, glaucoma, and cataracts.

48. Tip: Take your time when choosing what to eat when eating out, and don't be afraid to ask how the food is prepared. Being a little picky at the dinner table may save you some discomfort later on.

49. Tip: It can be easy to forget your routine on the road. Before you begin traveling, try setting reminders in your phone to take your medication and supplements.

50. Famous People with IBD: Shannen Doherty, an American actress, producer, author, and television director known for her work in Little House on the Prairie, Heathers, Our House, Beverly Hills 90210, and Charmed.

51. Do you exercise daily?: If not, plan a walk today during your lunch break for roughly 20 minutes. A little exercise daily can go a long way to increasing energy levels and improving symptoms.

52. Famous People with IBD: David Garrard, an American football quarterback who has played for the Jacksonville Jaguars, Miami Dolphins and the New York Jets.

53. Tip: Talking to someone else with IBD can be a huge help to understanding symptoms and receiving support. You are not alone. See if there is a support group for your disease in your area; if not, think about starting one.

54. Famous People with IBD: Chris Conley, singer for Saves the Day.

55. Did you know?: It is common for adults to experience some lactose intolerance symptoms as they age. This is especially true in people with Crohn's. If you feel you are experiencing more bloating or gas than normal, try reducing your dairy intake to see if symptoms improve. You can also utilize the many lactase additive products available for people with lactose intolerance.

56. Tip: Learn the terms. Learning the terms that your doctor is using and what they are looking for will help you to ask more educated questions and can help to give you a feeling of control.

57. Famous People with IBD: James Morrison, English professional golfer.

58. Did you know?: Protein depletion is a common side effect of IBD. Some symptoms of protein depletion can be swelling, stunted growth, bone pain, and an absence of menstrual periods.

59. Tip: If you have a hard time with needles, try icing the area to reduce the pain or ask your doctor about a skin numbing agent such as lidocaine.

60. Famous People with IBD: Jim Myers, AKA: George "The Animal" Steele, Professional WWE Wrestler and WWE Hall Of Fame inductee.

61. Tip: If you are experiencing a sudden loss in appetite for more than 1 or 2 days, call your doctor immediately. Many times, loss of appetite is a symptom of a flare or a blockage. Addressing it early can reduce the risks of needing to take extreme measures.

62. Tip: If you are experiencing cramps or abdominal pain, try applying a warm compress to your abdomen and finding the most comfortable position possible. This may help to alleviate some discomfort.

63. Famous People with IBD: Beth Orton, a famous British singer/songwriter.

64. Tip: Anemia is common for people with IBD due to the body's inability to properly absorb Vitamin B12. If you are feeling weak, look pale, or have been experiencing losses of appetite, ask your doctor about being tested for anemia. Many times a simple monthly B-12 shot can help to solve this common problem.

65. Tip: Eat 5 smaller meals a day. If that isn't feasible, try eating 3 medium-sized meals and 2 small meals or snacks a day.

66. Tip: Slow down; eating quickly can add to the amount of air you swallow, which can cause more gas and force your digestive system to work harder. Remember, digestion starts with chewing. Why not give your gut as much help as possible?

67. Tip: Stay Social! Multiple studies have proven that staying social can help you to feel better, recover more quickly, and keep a positive outlook. Even if you don't feel like eating, just drinking tea or water can still keep you as a part of the social activity.

68. Tip: Whenever you are about to have a procedure done or receive a new medication, it is important to understand the reasons for it. Ask your doctor simple why, what and how questions such as "Why is this being done?"; "What should the expected benefit be?"; and "How will this help me?"

69. Did you know?: Some people with Crohn's may experience eye inflammation. This is less common but occurs most commonly during a flare. This should be reported to your doctor immediately upon occurrence.

70. Famous People with IBD: Rocker McCready, lead guitarist for Pearl Jam.

71. Did you know?: People with IBD have a higher chance of developing kidney stones. To help avoid kidney stones many doctors recommend maintaining a mostly-water drink intake and avoiding foods that are rich in oxalates such as tea, spinach, beets, and cola.

72. Did you know?: Canker sores inside the mouth are common in people with Crohn's and are usually more present during a flare. Ask your doctor about topical ointments that can be used for treatment.

73. Tip: Make it a game to find new and unusual foods that can help you to reach your nutritional goals. This can help expand your available menus and help to spice up the dinner table. Remember, introducing new foods should be done in a controlled manner and recorded to see if there are any negative effects.

74. Tip: Master a few simple relaxation techniques to reduce stress. As an example, Tai Chi includes many very simple low-impact relaxation techniques that can be used throughout the day in almost any environment.

75. Tip: When going out in public, carry a pack of tissues just in case the place you are visiting is not well stocked with toilet paper.

76. Did you know?: Adding supplements to your vitamin intake may help to stabilize your weight and give you added energy. This is because your body may not be able to absorb specific nutrients as easily as others. Since each case is different, discuss which supplements may be beneficial to you with your doctor.

77. Did you know?: Gallstones are more common in people with IBD due to the inability to properly absorb bile salts. The most common symptoms of gallstones are pain the lower or upper right hand part of the belly which can also migrate to the right upper back area.

78. Tip: Fat malabsorption is common in people with IBD and can cause foul smelling stools. Many times, simply reducing the amount of fatty foods in your diet can alleviate this problem.

79. The Mayo Clinic recommends 3 liters of water per day for men, and 2.2 liters per day for women. Tip: Find a water bottle that holds roughly 1 liter of water and drink 1 bottle in the morning, 1 bottle in the afternoon, and 1 bottle at night.

80. Did you know?: Most doctors agree that fast food isn't necessarily all bad for IBD patients. However, try to choose healthy options off the menu and avoid high fat foods, which can aggravate symptoms.

81. Tip: Don't skip taking any of your medications, don't increase dosage and don't try to make up missed dosses. If you accidentally miss a scheduled dosage time or think you need a higher dose call your doctor and ask what should be done.

82. Tip: Lean proteins like chicken, fish and seafood are much more easily digestible than proteins from beef or pork, and they can be cooked almost any way you want.

83. Did you know?: Some doctors recommend getting tested for allergies to food and to regional allergens, as allergens exacerbate or even trigger symptoms. However, some medications cause specific allergy tests to be ineffective. Check with your doctor before having any allergy tests performed.

84. Did you know?: Protein is your body's main "repair" material. Try to incorporate at least two main sources of protein into your daily diet to help your body help itself.

85. Did you know?: Night sweats are a good clue as to whether or not your condition is under control. If you are commonly experiencing night sweats, it probably isn't. Let your doctor know if you are experiencing common occurrences of night sweats.

86. Tip: Eggs are a great source of easily digestible protein and can help make a great meal, even during a flare.

87. Did you know? Too much gut bacteria can be a bad thing. Some gut bacteria in large quantities can prevent the proper absorption of vitamins and can even produce toxic chemicals that can damage the intestinal lining. With this in mind, consult your doctor prior to starting any probiotics.

88. Tip: When planning to travel for an extended time (more than 1 week), notify your doctor and ask him or her to recommend a doctor in the location to which you will be traveling. This can help put your mind at ease, and it is a good safety measure.

89. Tip: To avoid aggravating symptoms, avoid eating at least 2 hours before going to bed. If that's not possible, go for a 20-minute walk before bed to aid your body's digestion.

90. Tip: It is usually a good idea to avoid foods that are highly acidic, such as 100 percent juice drinks, acid tomato sauces, coffee and sodas. The acid in these drinks can irritate the bowels and exacerbate symptoms.

91. Did you know?: Peanut butter and other nut butters are a great source of protein and can help if you have a craving for nuts. Make sure you only choose smooth nut butters, as others are more difficult to digest.

92. Tip: Antidiarrheal drugs can be beneficial for IBD patients; however, it is important to not become dependent or overuse them. Overuse can lead to an impacted colon, especially during a flare.

93. Famous People with IBD: Al Geiberger, a former professional American golfer who has won 11 PGA Tour tournaments.

94. Tip: Stick to a set daily routine in order to reduce stress and overcome the "blah" days. Keep a planner or set activities in your phone.

95. Did You Know?: Dwight D. Eisenhower, the United States' 34th President, was diagnosed with Crohn's and underwent surgery just 9 months after heart surgery. After surgery he was back in office and performing his duty within just 5 days!

96. Tip: If you don't want to take medication in a pill bottle to public places or work, try using a mint tin.

97. Tip: If you have children or are having a hard time explaining your disease to someone, try drawing a diagram to explain how it affects you. This also helps if you have a child with IBD and need to explain how taking their medication can help them.

98. Did you know?: An illness in the family can sometimes disrupt the way we communicate and interact with each other. Some IBD patients and their families have utilized family therapists who provide a safe, open environment to come to terms with the disease and establish communication.

99. Did you know?: Gummy or chewable vitamins absorb more readily into your system? Try switching to a gummy or chewable such as One-A-Day gummies.

100. Tip: If you're having a hard time feeling finished during a BM, try moving your upper body in a circular or figure-eight pattern while sitting upright. This should help to get anything left moving and ensure completion.

101. Tip: Traveling can increase chances for a flare. Maintaining a regular diet and medication schedule can help ensure an enjoyable trip.

NOTES

Made in the USA
Middletown, DE
06 August 2015